The Health Revolution in Cuba

Special Publication
Institute of Latin American Studies
The University of Texas at Austin

The Health Revolution in Cuba

by Sergio Díaz-Briquets

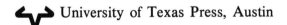 University of Texas Press, Austin

Library of Congress Cataloging in Publication Data

Díaz-Briquets, Sergio.
The health revolution in Cuba.

(Special publication)
Bibliography: p.
Includes index.
1. Mortality—Cuba—History. 2. Cuba—Statistics, Vital—
History. 3. Public health—Cuba—History. I. Title. II. Series:
Special publication (University of Texas at Austin.
Institute of Latin American Studies)
HB1379.D52 1983   304.6'4'097291   82-10865
ISBN 0-292-75071-4

Requests for permission to reproduce material from
this work should be sent to:
Permissions
University of Texas Press
P. O. Box 7819
Austin, Texas 78712

To my parents, Alberto and Amelia, and to my sister, Alina

Contents

Preface   xv

1. Introduction   3

2. The Secular Trend of Mortality in Cuba   11

3. The Premodern Period and the Initial Mortality Decline   25

4. The Context of the Mortality Decline in the First Half of the Twentieth Century   35

5. The Mortality Decline in Havana, 1901-1953   53

6. The Decline of Mortality from Specific Causes   67

7. The Mortality Decline in Cuba after 1953   103

8. Summary and Conclusions   119

Appendix 1: Evaluation of the Data   133

Appendix 2: Adjustments in the Data   145

Appendix 3: Sources and Evaluation of the Life Tables for Havana and Cuba   153

Appendix 4: Classifications of Causes of Death   167

Appendix 5: Statistical Appendix   173

Notes   195

Bibliography of Sources Not Cited in Text   221

Index   223

Tables

1. Decadal Average Crude Death Rates, City of Havana   12
2. Estimated Crude Death Rates by Province   15
3. Estimated Life Expectancies at Birth, Both Sexes Combined   19
4. Estimated Life Expectancies for Selected Latin American Countries, Both Sexes Combined   22
5. Cause-Specific Death Rates for Certain Infectious Diseases, City of Havana   30
6. Distribution of Dwellings by Type of Human-Waste Disposal Facility   42
7. Distribution of Dwellings by Type of Water-Supply System   43
8. Literacy of the Population over Ten Years of Age   45
9. Percentage of Cuba's Total Population Residing in Urban Areas, in Municipality of Havana, and in Metropolitan Havana   46
10. Population per Physician   50
11. Annual Death Rates per 1,000 Population, by Sex and Age, City of Havana   54
12. Age Group Contribution to Total Decline in Death Rate, Both Sexes Combined, City of Havana   55
13. Age Distribution of Population, Both Sexes Combined, City of Havana   56
14. Age-Sex-Standardized Cause-Specific Death Rates, Municipality of Havana   58
15. Contribution of Each Cause-Group or Cause of Death to Mortality Decline, City of Havana   60
16. Mortality Declines for Each Cause-Group as Percentage of Total Decline from All Causes, Municipality of Havana, 1907-1953   64
17. Declines in Age-Sex-Standardized Cause-Specific Death Rates, Municipality of Havana   70

18. Deaths Attributed to Malaria, Measles, and Smallpox   78

19. Regional Distribution of Hospital Beds   107

20. Distribution of Sanitary Facilities   108

21. Births and Deaths Occurring in Hospitals   110

22. Life Expectancies at Birth   111

23. Cause-Specific Death Rates for Selected American Countries, circa 1970   114

24. Estimated Life Expectancies at Birth for Selected Western Hemisphere Nations   116

25. Trends in Life Expectancy at Birth   120

26. Stages and Determinants of Cuba's Mortality Transition   127

27. Revisions of International List of Causes of Death Used by Cuban Statistical Service   135

28. Collver's Estimates of Completeness of Death and Birth Registration, Cuba   137

29. Estimated and Enumerated Population, 1 January 1953   138

30. Comparative Death Statistics and Estimated Completeness of Death Registration, 1948   139

31. Estimated and Official Crude Death Rates, 1900-1950   140

32. Estimated and Official Crude Death Rates, 1943-1953   141

33. Population, Number of Registered Deaths, and Crude Death Rates   143

34. Percentage of National Total of Registered Deaths and of Total Population   143

35. City of Havana Population as Percentage of Municipality of Havana Population   146

36. Age Distributions for Death Statistics, Municipality of Havana   150

37. Percentage of Distribution of Male Population over Age Five, Municipality of Havana   151

38. Age Distribution of Foreign-Born White Males   158

39. Estimated Life Expectancy at Birth and Absolute and Average Yearly Gains   161

40. Sex Differentials in Life Expectancy, Female over Male   162

41. Estimated Crude Death Rates, City of Havana   173

42. Life Tables, Municipality of Havana, 1901   174

43. Life Tables, Municipality of Havana, 1907   175
44. Life Tables, Municipality of Havana, 1919   176
45. Life Tables, Municipality of Havana, 1931   177
46. Life Tables, Municipality of Havana, 1943   178
47. Life Tables, Municipality of Havana, 1953   179
48. Life Tables, Cuba, 1919-1931   180
49. Life Tables, Cuba, 1931-1943   181
50. Life Tables, Cuba, 1952-1954   182
51. Life Tables, Cuba, 1970   183
52. Absolute Number of Deaths by Selected Causes, City of Havana   184
53. Age-Sex-Standardized Cause-Specific Death Rates, Municipality of Havana   185
54. Absolute Number of Deaths by Groups of Causes, Municipality of Havana   186
55. Absolute Number of Deaths by Groups of Causes, Cuba   189
56. Per Capita Consumption of Rice, Canned and Dry Milk, and Insecticides, Cuba   192

Figures

1. Estimated Crude Death Rates, City of Havana   14
2. Standardized and Crude Death Rates, City of Havana, Census Years   17
3. Crude and Cause-Specific Death Rates for Certain Infectious Diseases, City of Havana   29
4. Cuban Per Capita Income in Actual and Real Dollars   39
5. Cuban National Income, Exports, and Imports   40
6. Per Capita Consumption of Rice, Five-Year Moving Averages   49
7. Per Capita Consumption of Insecticides, Five-Year Moving Averages   49
8. Deaths Attributed to Respiratory Tuberculosis   71
9. Deaths Attributed to Other Infectious and Parasitic Diseases   74
10. Deaths Attributed to Malignant and Benign Tumors   84
11. Deaths Attributed to Cardiovascular Diseases   86
12. Deaths Attributed to Influenza, Pneumonia, and Bronchitis   88
13. Deaths Attributed to Diarrhea, Gastritis, and Enteritis   90
14. Deaths Attributed to Certain Degenerative Diseases   92
15. Deaths Attributed to Complications of Pregnancy   94
16. Deaths Attributed to Certain Diseases of Infancy   96
17. Deaths Attributed to Accidents and Violence   98
18. Deaths Attributed to All Other and Unknown Causes   99
19. Female q_x Curves from 1925 Cuban Life Table and from Regional Model Life-Tables   157
20. Female q_x Curves from 1937 Cuban Life Table and from Regional Model Life-Tables   160
21. Estimated Life Expectancy at Birth and at Selected Ages, Both Sexes Combined   164
22. Life-Table Death Rates (q_x), Both Sexes Combined, 1953   165

Preface

One of the most important developments shaping the course of civilization during the last two centuries has been the world-wide revolution in health and mortality. Conditions favoring better health have emerged and radical changes in mortality patterns have led to substantial gains in average longevity. In many countries of the world a child born today can expect to live more than seventy years, nearly three times as long as those born before the beginning of the health revolution—circa 1750. This dramatic departure from mankind's ancient relation to nature can only be compared to that associated with the Industrial Revolution.

What brought about the health and mortality revolution is still subject to a great deal of conjecture. By evaluating secular changes observed in Cuba's mortality record, I have tried to establish how and under what conditions the revolution manifested itself there. Although inexact in many ways, this reconstructed mortality record provides a revealing view of the country's past, particularly the statistics of death-by-cause. Despite their shortcomings, these statistics constitute one of the most reliable and unbiased indicators of those developments in society-at-large that determine changes in health and mortality. To the extent that the mortality statistics capture the effects of those developments, the statistics provide a unique historical perspective on the nature of social change. We can relate medical, public health, social, economic, and political developments known to have occurred in the country to changes in cause-specific mortality. We can interpret the nature of these changes, in turn, in light of scientific evidence concerning the prevention and cure of specific diseases. Mortality statistics, therefore, are a useful, if imperfect vehicle through which we can evaluate different features of a country's history.

In few other countries can such an analysis be as productive as in Cuba, given the highly politicized interpretation of Cuba's history since the 1959 socialist revolution. A great deal of controversy surrounds the study of the levels of social and economic development that prerevolutionary Cuba achieved. Unfortunately, many of those who participate in the debate—on both sides—rely on impressionistic interpretations to substantiate their views. For most of my life I have followed this debate and I hope that this study contributes toward a better understanding of twentieth-century Cuba. Like many other Cuban-born researchers who have studied Cuban society from abroad, I have always been conscious of potential personal biases arising from my ideological preferences. As a result, I have gone to great lengths to interpret the evidence as objectively and as carefully as possible.

This study constitutes an expanded and revised version of my doctoral dissertation in demography at the University of Pennsylvania; thus the study benefited to an incalculable extent from the intellectual environment provided by the faculty and students of the Population Studies Center there. My greatest debt is to the late Professor John D. Durand who, as my dissertation committee chairman and a towering intellect, greatly influenced my research strategy. The multidisciplinary perspective that constitutes the very essence of this study is a direct result of Professor Durand's own approach to socioeconomic-demographic research. His patience and assistance as a skillful, encouraging, and sympathetic mentor during and after my graduate studies will always be gratefully remembered.

Professors Richard A. Easterlin and Etienne van de Walle, also committee members, gave me invaluable insights and assistance concerning many research issues. Their experience with the interpretive problems associated with the use of historical data allowed me to overcome many conceptual and technical hurdles. Other members of the Population Studies Center, in particular Professors Ann Miller and Edward P. Hutchinson, were invariably helpful.

Joan M. Herold, a good and trusted friend and fellow student, endured my recurrent "research moods" and influenced the direction of this study more times than I can remember. Rolando E. Bonachea, a life-long friend, helped me retain a realistic outlook when most needed and provided the spark that led me to undertake this study. Armando Chapelli has, over the years, contributed to my mental health in more ways than I can remember. Other friends and colleagues in and out of the University of Pennsylvania were also helpful and often provided an escape from the most tedious and least gratifying aspects of research. Among these I would especially like to thank Olivier Blanc, Lillian Cabrera, Teofilus Fadayomi, John McHenry, and Virginia Schofield for their tolerance and friendship. Lourdes Flor-Lachapelle and Jorge Pérez-López provided me with various sources of information used in the study.

My parents and sister, and my uncle Rafael gave me all of the affection and moral support that I needed.

The revised version of the original study was greatly improved by the comments and suggestions of Professors Michael E. Conroy, Eileen C. Crimmins, Lisandro Pérez, and Samuel H. Preston, who reviewed the manuscript.

I am also grateful to Kathy Schnabel, Lydia Christaldi, Don Goldstein, Susan O'Connor, Randi Reinis, Judy Robinson, and especially Pam Butcher and Lisa C. Olson who helped me with various chores associated with the manuscript's preparation. The staff of the Hispanic Division of the Library of Congress was most helpful during my research.

Some of the materials included in the monograph were published under the title "Determinants of Mortality Transition in Developing Countries Before and After the Second World War: Some Evidence from Cuba," in *Population Studies* 35, no. 3 (November 1981).

The study's original research and completion of my graduate work were supported by a three-year fellowship on population and development, granted by the Population Studies Center and financed by the Rockefeller Foundation. Partial support from a grant by the Ford Foundation to the center was used in an earlier revision of the study. Of course, I alone am responsible for the conclusions.

The Health Revolution in Cuba

1. Introduction

Mortality statistics are increasingly recognized as one of the more reliable and accessible indicators of the well-being of a country. They reflect how a population is affected by public health, medical, social, economic, environmental, and political conditions. As such, we may regard mortality measures and trends as a window on the welfare of a nation: they indicate what is being accomplished in the process of social and economic development.

The purpose of this study is to analyze how selected factors have contributed to the long-term trend of mortality decline in Cuba during approximately the last one hundred years. From the beginning of the twentieth century to the mid-1970s, Cuba made the transition from a dismal mortality regime to one comparable to those found in the more economically advanced nations. The benefits we may gain from an understanding of this mortality transformation extend beyond the narrower confines of a country's history and beyond the specialized interests of disciplines such as demography and public health.

An analysis of the Cuban mortality experience can be especially fruitful in understanding the causes of mortality change in many parts of the world. Cuba has comparatively extensive and revealing demographic, social, and economic records, by developing-country standards. Cuba's size, the relative homogeneity of its population, and its geographical isolation have been important factors in the preservation of useful import/export records. Analysis of Cuban mortality records also permits inferences about a wide range of events in Cuban society and an investigation of how the country was affected by developments within and outside its borders. And such analysis can help find answers to questions more easily understood with a statistical base, for example, the levels of social and economic development of Cuba before and after the socialist revolution.

Since the revolution, a highly emotional and politically and ideologically motivated controversy has raged about the country's republican past. Official revolutionary-government sources and many defenders of the regime abroad tend to portray prerevolutionary Cuba as a country of overwhelming social and economic injustices, while their opponents, vocal exiles in particular, tend to exaggerate the achievements of the Cuba of bygone days. This study points out the weaknesses and strengths of both positions.

The performance of prerevolutionary Cuban governments in promoting social justice, as evidenced by the mortality data analyzed here, was relatively successful, compared with most other developing countries. A life expectancy of over sixty years attained by the late 1950s testifies to that fact. This does not imply, however, that social and economic differentials in access to public health and other life essentials were not significant. Social class and rural-urban differentials most definitely were present. The revolution, by reducing these inequities, created the conditions that have allowed Cuba to achieve a very favorable life expectancy, closer to those found in developed countries than to those prevalent in most of the developing world. Unfortunately, this achievement has been accomplished at high political and social costs that many consider excessive.

As the study reveals, certain critical political events in Cuban history provided the junctures at which important mortality changes began to take place. The first of these events occurred at the turn of the twentieth century, when Cuba was occupied by American military forces for three years, following the Spanish-American War. At that time, extensive sanitary reforms were instituted in the country, which resulted in Cuba's first recorded and long-lasting improvement of mortality (largely due to the reduction of epidemic outbreaks). This reduction made possible sustained mortality declines in later years. This was also a period in which Cuba's powerful northern neighbor began to influence Cuba's mortality transition. Sixty years later, in 1959, another political event, the socialist revolution, appears to have created the necessary conditions for further improvement of mortality, at a time when mortality was already quite low.

Economic factors also played an important part in Cuba's mortality decline. In this regard the Cuban experience offers a rare opportunity to study the interrelationship between economic and demographic events. The historical evidence strongly suggests that the mortality trend was highly sensitive to the ups and downs of the Cuban economy during the first half of the twentieth century: when economic conditions were favorable, mortality declined; when the economy deteriorated during the 1930s, the mortality trend suffered accordingly. But during the 1960s mortality levels improved, even though the economy had entered a long-lasting period of deterioration.

In Cuba, as in other developing countries, mortality declines partially resulted from the gradual sanitary and medical breakthroughs that originated in more-developed countries. For example, Cuba recorded a dramatic decline in mortality following the Second World War, but contrary to what has been claimed for other tropical countries, malaria control appears to have played only a minor role. Of overwhelming significance in this decline was the response of other causes of death (such as influenza and pneumonia) to modern drugs.

We can reach a fuller understanding of the impact on Cuban society of Cuba's mortality transition by placing the country's experience in an international perspective. Modern mortality decline, of course, is not unique to Cuba. It constitutes one of the most significant events ever to have affected humanity, since it has led to an unprecedented increase in the growth rate and size of the world's population during the last two centuries.

In the absence of migration, population growth results from the difference between the number of births and the number of deaths. Since declines in birth rates, when observed, have usually lagged behind declines in death rates, the rate of population increase has accelerated, following the appearance of modern mortality conditions, in most countries. We can fully appreciate the enormous impact of mortality changes on the size of the world's population only when we realize that sustained mortality declines have disrupted the historically established balance between mortality and fertility that maintained population growth-rates at low levels for thousands of years. It took mankind a million years to attain a population of close to 8 million, from when man first appeared on Earth to the time of the agricultural revolution (sometime around 8000 B.C.). Population growth then accelerated, but by the beginning of the Christian Era the size of the world's population was only near 300 million.[1] According to John D. Durand, the population of the world probably did not exceed 800 million by 1750. However, by 1900, the world's population had more than doubled, to about 1.7 billion. Since that time the pace of population growth has further accelerated, with population reaching nearly 4 billion in 1975.[2] Most current projections suggest that by the year 2000, world population will increase by nearly 50 percent, to about 6 billion.[3]

Mortality declines have almost always been followed by fertility declines, although a few exceptions to this general trend have been observed.[4] Yet in most countries where populations of European origin predominate, and in many countries in Asia and Latin America, declining mortality has preceded declining fertility. The regularity of this pattern had led students of population processes to formulate a theory of demographic transition.[5] In essence, the demographic transition theory summarizes empirical evidence that indicates that human populations during socioeconomic development move from a situation of high birth and death rates to one of low birth and death rates. During the early stages of the demographic transition, improvements in socioeconomic conditions or advances in sanitary or medical practices induce the beginning of a sustained mortality decline.

Norms favoring high birth rates evolved throughout a long history of high mortality and are resistant to change. Population growth accelerates during this phase. Eventually, modernizing influences begin to erode high-fertility norms, and the birth rate also begins a sustained decline. At some point, a new equilibrium is reached at which birth and death rates attain similarly low levels. As this happens, low historical levels of population growth rates are achieved again.

Demographers understand fairly well the general features of the history of world-wide transition from high to low mortality. At some point during the eighteenth century a secular trend of mortality decline began in northern and western Europe. The mortality decline gradually spread to eastern and southern Europe and to other countries populated primarily by people of European ancestry. Sometime after the beginning of the twentieth century mortality declines got underway in developing countries. The phenomenon became almost universal following the Second World War, although even at the present time, some countries in Africa and Asia are just entering their mortality transition.

The onset of mortality decline has extended over more than two centuries, and whenever it has appeared it has followed a similar pattern. Before the transition begins, mortality is characterized by violent and unpredictable fluctuations. As the transition begins, those fluctuations begin to disappear and the trend becomes more gradual. The intensity and speed of the decline varies from country to country, according to the historical period and the level of socioeconomic development at which the mortality decline originated.

In European countries the pace of mortality decline was very slow, since it was brought about by step-by-step improvements in socioeconomic conditions and by a gradual accumulation of medical and sanitary knowledge. In contrast, mortality declines in many developing countries have been abrupt and have resulted in relatively low mortality levels after only a few years, rather than over decades.

Abdel Omran differentiates three basic models of mortality decline, according to the time at which the decline began and to the rate of decline.[6] The classical, or western model summarizes the experience of European countries, in which mortality slowly declined over many decades as socioeconomic conditions improved. The accelerated model also corresponds to a gradual process of mortality change, but compressed over a shorter period of time (Japan is a classic example). The contemporary, or delayed model describes the recent and rapid mortality declines observed in most developing countries. Frequently, these sudden and rapid mortality declines have taken place in the absence of socioeconomic change and have been produced by the importation of chemical and medical measures originating in the developed countries. Some of the most dramatic declines in death rates, produced by the importation of disease-fighting measures from advanced countries, took place in countries like Sri Lanka (Ceylon) and Guyana (British Guiana), where massive amounts of residual insecticides were utilized after the Second World War to destroy malaria-producing mosquitoes.[7]

Controversy concerning the specific mechanisms responsible for the reduction of mortality rates during modern times centers on the improvements that took place during the early stages of this trend. Some researchers postulate that the start of the mortality decline corresponds to the gradual change in conditions that led to the catastrophic mortality common in the premodern era. These conditions were, for the most part, malnutrition, famine, and epidemic disease. Improvements in agricultural techniques, the introduction of new crops, improved means of transportation, and other developments associated with the beginning of the Industrial Revolution in Europe significantly improved the availability of food and provided for a richer diet. These developments, along with favorable climatic changes, rising income levels, and a possible reduction in the virulence of some infectious organisms contributed to less-frequent severe mortality peaks, a precondition for further mortality declines.[8]

The effects of medical advances on the mortality trend, at least until the twentieth century, appear to have been only moderate. Thomas McKeown, after a careful review of medical and statistical evidence, concludes, in one of the most influential assessments of the impact of medical progress on mortality, that "it is unlikely that immunization or therapy had a significant effect on mortality from infectious diseases before the twentieth century."[9] The exception to this, McKeown notes, is the moderate effect of vaccination against smallpox, during the 1848-54 period. This categorical conclusion is not, however, accepted by other observers, who claim that inoculation against smallpox did play a very significant role in the early mortality declines in Europe, specifically in England and Wales.[10] Neither is it accepted by those who believe that medical advances made minor but significant contributions to declining mortality before the beginning of the twentieth century.[11] By the latter part of the nineteenth century the sanitary reforms associated with the acceptance of the germ theory of disease and the development of a wide range of public health measures intensified the established mortality-decline trend begun earlier largely because of socioeconomic changes and improvements in diet.

Less controversy surrounds the variables that have led to a continuation of mortality declines in developed countries in recent decades and to the rapid onset of mortality changes in the developing world. Medical and sanitary advances, including innovations in chemotherapy and immunization against disease, have clearly played a dominant role. Other factors, such as economic growth, nutrition level, income distribution, and use of insecticides, have also been involved to various extents in different countries. There is no consensus, however, as to the relative weights of these forces in mortality declines: studies dealing with one region or country tend to attach more importance to some variables than to others. Undoubtedly, the diversity of findings may be explained partly by the varying social, economic, sanitary, and historical conditions of the countries considered.

Differences in the pace of mortality decline between countries that entered their transitions long ago or more recently suggest that economic conditions, broadly defined, were the most significant factors in the initiation of the modern mortality era. However, since many events likely to affect mortality trends were taking place, and since economic growth and mortality declines occurred concurrently, it is difficult to isolate cause-and-effect relationships. Some analysts, such as McKeown and associates, in their interpretation of the mortality decline in England and Wales, and in other European countries, tacitly assume that economic conditions were improving as mortality was declining.[12] Students of more-recent mortality declines in certain developing countries postulate that mortality declines have taken place almost completely independent of economic improvements.[13] Eduardo Arriaga and Kingsley Davis, in an examination of mortality data from Latin American countries, find evidence indicating that the link between socioeconomic improvements and mortality declines has weakened over the past fifty years, as factors exogenous to a country's socioeconomic conditions have begun to acquire increasing importance.[14] In an examination of the changing relationship between income levels (as a proxy measure for advances in socioeconomic conditions) and mortality, Samuel H. Preston concludes that "mortality has not become progressively dissociated from standards of living at a moment in time." What has occurred, he suggests, is that the relationship between mortality measures and income has shifted upward, since improvements in medical and sanitary know-how permit lower mortality levels at lower levels of income and socioeconomic development.[15]

A number of structural transformations in the patterns of mortality by age and by cause of death accompany the process of declining mortality. Although differences in the incidence of mortality by age are evident at all levels of mortality,

the typical age-specific mortality curve in countries of high mortality is roughly *U*-shaped, the left-hand value of the "U" representing the high mortality of infancy and the right-hand value corresponding to the mortality of old age. As expectation of life increases, infant mortality falls much faster than mortality at old age, and the curve therefore assumes more of a *J*-shape. In addition, its base becomes broader, indicating that low mortality rates extend over a larger number of age groups.[16]

A pronounced structural change also occurs in the pattern of mortality by cause of death, as countries make the transition from high to low death rates. At high levels of mortality, deaths produced by infectious causes dominate the death distribution. As mortality declines, their incidence is reduced significantly, as degenerative diseases gain importance. In their analysis of mortality changes by cause of death (with data from 165 populations at different levels of mortality), Samuel Preston and Verne E. Nelson found that nearly 60 percent of the decline in death rates during the mortality transition can be attributed to drops in mortality from infectious diseases, distributed as follows: influenza, pneumonia, and bronchitis (25 percent); respiratory tuberculosis (10 percent); diarrheal diseases (10 percent); other infectious and parasitic diseases (15 percent). Cardiovascular deaths, many of which have an infectious origin, were found to contribute a further 25 percent to mortality decline. One striking feature of this structural change is that the relative contribution of each of these groups of causes of death is fairly similar, regardless of the initial and final levels of mortality.[17]

Keeping this historical perspective in mind, I will evaluate the Cuban mortality experience against the background of the world-wide mortality transition. The Cuban records clarify many of the features of the world-wide transition, especially in developing countries, and also capture, if only in a limited sense, how Cuba's process of social and economic development has influenced the well-being of its population over the span of a century. Chapter 2 establishes the secular trend of mortality in Cuba from the late-nineteenth century to the present and compares the Cuban experience to that of other Latin American countries; Chapter 3 assesses the causes of high mortality during the nineteenth century and factors behind the beginning of the modern mortality decline; Chapter 4 examines some political, economic, social, and medical developments associated with the mortality decline during the first half of this century. Chapters 5 and 6 analyze mortality trends from 1901 to 1953, in terms of changes in mortality by age and by cause of death. These two chapters are mainly based on evidence from the City of Havana, although data from the rest of Cuba were incorporated whenever possible. The results discussed in Chapter 5 closely agree with the international evidence summarized in the Introduction; readers not interested in the finer demographic points of the study may want to bypass this chapter. Chapter 6 relates the changes in mortality by cause to the historical developments reviewed in Chapter 4 and identifies the main determinants of mortality changes between 1901 and 1953. The chapter concludes with an assessment of the implications of analysis of mortality statistics for understanding how changing conditions during the first half of this century affected the welfare of the Cuban people. Chapter 7 examines the determinants of the mortality changes that have occurred in Cuba since the revolution, and the final chapter presents a summary and the conclusions that emerge from the study. The appendices evaluate the quality of the demographic data used in the study, describe some of the adjustments made to the data, and present some of the statistical material—demographic and economic—discussed in the text.

2. The Secular Trend of Mortality in Cuba

A description of the secular trend of mortality in Cuba must rely on fragmentary and at times inadequate data. The limitations of data dictate the measures we can use and how far we can carry the analysis. In some periods, we can compute only crude death rates for limited areas.[1] In others, we can supplement the crude rates by calculating standardized rates and life tables.[2] For certain periods, when death registration was very deficient, we must fill gaps by estimating gross tendencies by means of the application of nonconventional techniques. These techniques produce life-table measures by comparing age structures recorded in consecutive census enumerations.[3] By combining different sets of measures, we can obtain a fairly detailed view of the trend of mortality decline in the country.

The amounts of available data define three distinct periods. Most of the data prior to 1902 are concerned exclusively with the experience of the City of Havana, although some additional sources allow limited generalizations about the mortality conditions of the country as a whole. From 1902 through 1953, a more complete, although still weak, statistical record permits a more refined treatment. During this fifty-two-year interval, data are available not only for Havana, but also for the country as a whole, albeit with many limitations. Six censuses, the first in 1899, the last in 1953, serve as a basis for a wide range of estimates. For the years since 1953, a more limited amount of statistical material exists and provides data at an aggregate level for the whole country. A dearth of data is evident for the late 1950s and early 1960s, but data availability improved significantly by around 1970 (the high point for this period is the 1970 census).

Mortality Trend by Means of Crude Death Rate Estimates

Some questionable but highly suggestive data for Havana and other areas of Cuba, dating from before the twentieth century, indicate premodern mortality conditions. Decadal average crude death rates for the City of Havana (shown in table 1) demonstrate that throughout the nineteenth century, the mortality trend was characterized by violent and unpredictable fluctuations and at times reached exceedingly high levels. In practically every interval during the period, major outbreaks of epidemic diseases were recorded and probably accounted for most of the period-to-period fluctuations.

Table 1
Decadal Average Crude Death Rates, City of Havana

Decade	Crude Death Rate	Recorded Epidemics and Wars
1801-1810	38.0	
1811-1820	46.7	Yellow fever, 1816-1820
1821-1830	36.2	
1831-1840	32.2	Cholera, 1833-1836
1841-1850	23.3	Yellow fever, 1844
1851-1860	26.2	Asiatic cholera, 1850-1854
1861-1870	42.0	Asiatic cholera, 1867-1868
		Yellow fever, 1861
1871-1880	45.0	Yellow fever, 1873-1877
		Smallpox, 1871-1872; 1874-1875; 1878-1881
		Ten Years' War, 1868-1878
1881-1890	34.2	Smallpox, 1887-1888
1891-1900	43.8	Yellow fever, 1885-1898
		Smallpox, 1891; 1894-1898
		War of Independence, 1895-1898

Sources: Adapted from Junta Nacional del Censo, *Censo de la República de Cuba—1919*, Havana, no date, p. 258; and Hugh Thomas, *Cuba: The Pursuit of Freedom* (New York: Harper & Row, 1971), p. 284.

These figures are revealing, but they may not convey the true situation, since their credibility is in doubt. From what we know about death registration in general, and specifically about the past reliability of these statistical records, it seems likely that there was an underregistration of deaths. Similar reservations must be made regarding the reliability of the population data used in computing the crude death rates. What we can infer with certainty from this series is that mortality was very high and that it fluctuated greatly, owing to epidemic diseases.

Evidence from other parts of the country indicates that the situation

elsewhere was not very different from that of Havana. Guy Bourdé, a
French historical demographer who has recently done work on the evaluation of Cuban ecclesiastical records in areas outside of Havana, found
similarly high mortality and the characteristic swings in the death rates.[4] In
his study of late-eighteenth century and nineteenth century parish records of
Santa María del Rosario (located thirty kilometers from the center of
Havana), he estimated crude death rates that at their highest levels rivaled
those estimated for Havana.

The detailed demographic record that has been preserved for the City of
Havana since before 1880 allows the estimation of a yearly series of death
rates from that date to 1953. These yearly crude death rates are depicted
graphically in figure 1 (the values are presented in Appendix 4). There were
erratic fluctuations of the rates between 1880 and 1900. The extreme peak
between about 1895 and 1898 is partly due to a brutal war (the Cuban War
of Independence), during which living conditions so deteriorated that famine
and pestilence became rampant (see table 2 for a fuller assessment of the
effect of the war on mortality in the country as a whole). Although these
rates reflect underregistration, as we can deduce from the very low values
prior to 1895, they show a remarkable upswing in the war years. During
those years, a Spanish expeditionary force of nearly 200,000 soldiers sent to
end the rebellion flooded the country. Moreover, rural inhabitants were
forced to concentrate in the heavily garrisoned urban areas, as part of a war
policy designed to deny popular support to the insurgent Cuban troops in the
field. Uncertainties regarding the magnitude of the "migratory" element
hamper the adjustment of the population figures on which the yearly rates for
Havana are based. Registration of deaths of transitory residents of the city,
in particular members of the Spanish expeditionary force and the rural
population forced to move to Havana, undoubtedly tend to inflate the rates.
Nevertheless, it is evident that a great increase in mortality occurred as
living conditions became chaotic. Sanitary standards deteriorated severely,
epidemic outbreaks became more violent and lethal, and military casualties
were in the tens of thousands. The country's population declined from about
1,800,000 to some 1,500,000 between 1895 and 1899, largely as a result of
the increased mortality, but also partly because of a decline in the birth rate.
According to Hugh Thomas, "Few nations had lost as high a proportion of
population in a war before that date."[5]

The occupation of the country by the United States Army in 1898, at the
close of the Spanish-American War, led almost immediately to a decline in
the death rate. Not only did the war cease, but radical sanitary measures
were instituted that practically wiped out certain epidemic diseases while
decreasing the incidence of other maladies.

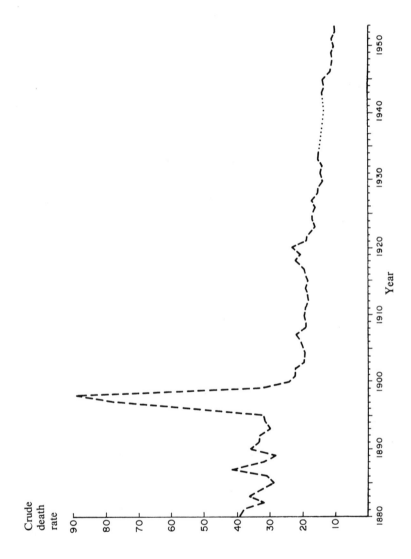

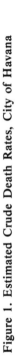

Figure 1. Estimated Crude Death Rates, City of Havana

Table 2
Estimated Crude Death Rates by Province

Year	Province						
	Cuba	Pinar del Río	Havana	Matanzas	Santa Clara	Cama-güey	Oriente
1890	17.2	8.0	36.2	25.9	22.0	16.5	11.2
1891	16.7	7.3	34.0	23.6	21.7	14.7	12.4
1892	17.1	7.5	33.8	27.2	22.0	14.3	10.6
1893	16.7	7.3	31.7	26.5	22.6	13.3	9.9
1894	12.6	7.5	30.7	—	22.4	12.9	10.1
1895	21.3	12.4	33.3	27.7	26.1	26.8	19.9
1896	35.1	39.8	51.9	43.6	40.1	28.7	30.2
1897	73.0	76.3	79.0	111.2	127.6	38.1	30.4
1898	68.3	75.5	91.0	84.1	113.3	32.6	36.8
1899	—	23.9	34.6	—	—	21.6	10.9

Source: United States War Department, *Report on the Census of Cuba—1899* (Washington, D.C., 1900), p. 718.

We may attribute subsequent fluctuations in the death rates observed in the chart to both short-term changes in the actual mortality levels and biases in the figures. For example, the increase in 1907 coincides with a second military occupation of Cuba by American forces, following a period of civil unrest. It is probable that under the military administration, the civil government functioned more effectively than it normally did, and the registration of deaths may have improved. An influenza epidemic also was recorded that year. The peak in 1918 was due to the world-wide influenza epidemic, an interpretation substantiated by inspection of the cause-of-death statistics. By 1920 the pandemic was over, yet, it was during this year that the highest crude death rate level during this century was reached. The statistics on international migration provide a credible explanation. It was during 1920 that the greatest number of international arrivals ever recorded in Cuba entered the country, nearly 175,000, or over double the average of the 1910-1925 period. Higher mortality among these immigrants than among the resident population at the time may have resulted in an excessively high death rate in 1920. Data on deaths by cause support this view (see Chapter 6). After 1920 the curve shows a gradual tendency to decline, except for minor fluctuations, until about 1945, when it declines steadily until about 1953.

Mortality Trend by Means of Estimates of Standardized Death Rates

Since changes in the age composition of the population affect the crude death rate level, it is advisable to eliminate compositional effects when studying mortality trends. We can accomplish this by standardizing different estimates of the death rate to a common age-structure. Figure 2 shows the age- and sex-standardized death rates at six censal years, and the age-standardized death rates for each sex (the estimated Havana population of 1901 was the standard used).[6] The standardized rates show a more pronounced decline than do the crude rates. From 1901 to 1919 the standardized rates remained fairly stable. From 1919 to 1931 a significant decline took place, which slowed considerably between 1931 and 1943, and then accelerated until 1953. The curve for the males shows a noticeable increase in 1919 (average of 1918, 1919, and 1920), quite consistent with the immigration that occurred at that time. In contrast, the female curve shows a slight lowering of the rate for that year. This difference may partly reflect poorer registration of female than of male deaths, but it is consistent with the heavy male domination of the migration stream,[7] although inconsistent with the effects of the influenza pandemic. With this exception, the male and female curves exhibit similar patterns, but the male rates are always higher than those of the females. Some reservations regarding the very rapid decline between 1919 and 1931 will be elaborated on later.

Mortality Trend by Means of Life-Table Estimates

We cannot obtain dependable death rates for most of the years under study for Cuba as a whole without extensive and questionable adjustments, since death registration outside principal urban centers was very deficient. It is possible, however, to describe the trend of declining mortality for the total Cuban population with life-table estimates. We can compare the Cuban life-table estimates with similar life-table values derived for the City of Havana at about the same dates to determine whether similar trends of declining mortality characterized the city and the country.

I have constructed a series of six life tables for Havana, 1901 to 1953, by relating the registered number of deaths in the city in or near census years to the population of the city enumerated in censuses (the 1899 enumerated population of Havana being projected to 1901). Students at the Centro Latinoamericano de Demografía (CELADE) in Santiago, Chile, have estimated life tables for the population of Cuba as a whole in the intercensal periods 1919-1931 and 1931-1943 and the years 1952-1954.[8] For the purpose of this study, I have extended their series of Cuban life-tables over

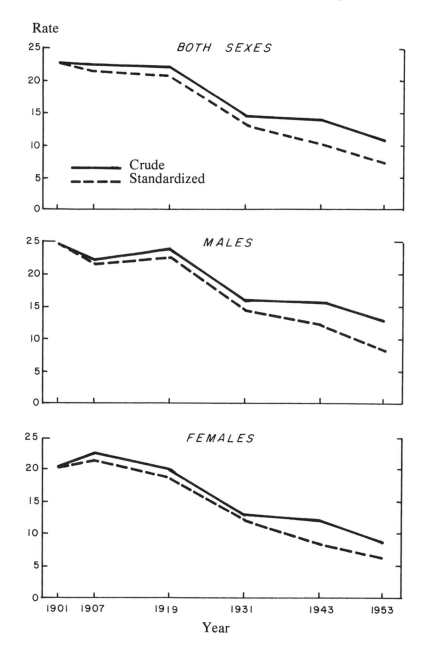

Figure 2. Standardized and Crude Death Rates, City of Havana, Census Years

the earlier decades of the century by means of estimates derived from the census statistics for the periods 1899-1909 and 1909-1919.[9] Henceforth, I shall refer to the period tables, for convenience, by the middle-year dates (1905 for 1899-1909, 1915 for 1909-1919, 1925 for 1919-1931, 1937 for 1931-1943, and 1953 for 1952-1954). An official Cuban statistical agency has made a life table for 1970 available.[10] On the basis of these life tables, others have interpolated more life tables to obtain mortality estimates for every five years from 1900 to 1950.

Table 3 summarizes life expectancy trends at birth (e_o) by all the available Havana and Cuba life tables for both sexes combined. The general pattern agrees with that observed in the crude and standardized death rates. In both Havana and Cuba the levels of life expectancy rise, slowly at first, but gain momentum in the later periods. For the 1920-1930 period, the Cuban life-table series shows a slower acceleration in the rate of gain in life expectancy than the Havana series for about the same dates. The actual gain in Cuba at the time was probably greater, since certain biases in the estimation of the 1925 life table appear to have understated the mortality decline (the biases are discussed in Appendix 3).

The Havana life tables show a pronounced mortality decline between 1919 and 1931. Evidence discussed later in this study strongly supports this interpretation; however, it should be noted that shortcomings in the data for this period may exaggerate somewhat the mortality decline between those two dates. A nationwide deterioration in the vital statistics registration system at the time of the Great Depression may also have spuriously magnified the mortality decline. (For a discussion of these problems, see Appendix 3.)

Between 1925 and 1937 the Cuba series shows large gains in life expectancy, in contrast with the Havana data for 1931-1943, which show comparatively small gains. Since this period involved several different mortality experiences, as well as biases in some life tables, a definitive interpretation of the trends is extremely difficult. However, a probable overestimation of mortality in Cuba for 1925 and 1937 (see Appendix 3) would account for some of the differences the Havana and Cuba series exhibit in the trends for the 1930s and 1940s. We should also consider the likelihood that the rest of Cuba trailed Havana in mortality reduction during much of this period because of marked differences in health facilities, sanitary conditions, and general amenities.

The estimates for the 1937-1953 period for Cuba, which correspond to the 1943-1953 intercensal period for Havana, indicate a significant acceleration in the rate of gains in life expectancy for both. The Cuba data for the intercensal period of 1953 to 1970 (data are not available for Havana)

Table 3
Estimated Life Expectancies at Birth, Both Sexes Combined

Year	Estimated Life Expectancy (Years)	
	Havana	Cuba
1900		33.2[e]
1901	37.2[a]	
1905	36.4[a]	34.2[e]
1907	39.1[a]	
1910		35.3[e]
1915	37.2[a]	36.3[e]
1919	41.3[a]	
1920		37.4[e]
1925	39.2[b]	38.5[e]
1930		41.5[e]
1931	50.8[a]	
1935		44.6[e]
1937	46.4[b]	
1940		47.5[e]
1943	54.0[a]	
1945		51.0[e]
1950		55.8[e]
1953	62.7[a]	58.8[c]
1955		60.7[f]
1960		64.0[f]
1965		67.2[f]
1970	70.1[d]	70.0[f]
1980		71.8[g]

Sources: [a] Data from this study; [b] Rodolfo Mezquita, *Cuba: Estimación de la mortalidad por sexo. Tabla de vida para los períodos 1919-31 y 1931-43*, series C, no. 121 (Santiago, Chile: Centro Latinoamericano de Demografía, March 1970); [c] Fernando González Q. and Jorge Debasa, *Cuba: Evaluación y ajuste del censo de 1953 y las estadísticas de nacimientos y defunciones entre 1943 y 1958. Tabla de mortalidad por sexo, 1952-54*, series C, no. 124 (Santiago, Chile: Centro Latinoamericano de Demografía, 1970); [d] Junta Central de Planificación (JUCEPLAN), *La esperanza o expectativa de vida* (Havana: JUCEPLAN, 1974); [e] Elio Velásquez and Lázaro Toirao, *Cuba: Tablas de mortalidad estimadas por sexo, para los años calendarios terminados en cero y cinco durante el período 1900-1950*, Estudios Demográficos, series 1, no. 3 (Havana: University of Havana, July 1975); [f] Alfonso Farnos Morejón, *Cuba: Tablas de mortalidad estimadas por sexo. Período 1955-1970*, Estudios Demográficos, series 1, no. 8 (Havana: University of Havana, December 1976); [g] Centro Latinoamericano de Demografía (San José), and Dirección de Demografía (Cuba), "Proyección de la población cubana 1950-2000, nivel nacional: Metodología y resultados," Havana, August 1978.

Note: See Appendices 1, 2, and 3 for a description of the data used in computing some of the life tables, as well as for the evaluation of the life-table series.

suggest a continuation of the rapid increase, and CELADE suggests that the trend of mortality decline continues to the present. CELADE estimates a life expectancy of 71.8 years for Cuba in 1975-1980 and projects that it will rise to 72.5 years during 1980-1985.[11] If these estimated life-expectancy levels reflect reality, we can consider Cuba to be one of the developing countries with the lowest mortality rates in the world.

The Cuban Experience in the Latin American Context

We can compare the secular trend in life expectancy for Cuba with that of other Latin American countries. Eduardo Arriaga has estimated trends for seventeen countries in the region for years for which data were available. His estimates, interpolated to the beginning of each decade, are summarized in table 4. Similar estimates for Argentina and Buenos Aires are included at the bottom of this table. The Cuba and Havana estimates appear in table 3.

These data indicate that throughout the twentieth century Cuba led most other Latin American countries in life expectancy. At the beginning of the century only Argentina had a higher life expectancy than Cuba.[12] In fact, only Cuba, Argentina, and Costa Rica had reached a life expectancy of more than thirty years.[13] The unique position of Argentina is evident: by the early 1900s it had attained life expectancy levels that Cuba and a few other countries were to reach only by the Second World War. By World War II only Panama, Costa Rica, and Cuba had life expectancies of over forty years, with the latter two countries exceeding by approximately ten years the levels recorded for the rest of the region.

Following the Second World War, gains in life expectancy accelerated significantly world-wide. Relative differences between leading and lagging countries, however, remained, and in some cases became even greater. Differences in life expectancy between Costa Rica and Cuba, on the one hand, and countries such as Brazil, the Dominican Republic, and Nicaragua on the other, became greater than before. Argentina still retained its lead, although it seems that Cuba, Costa Rica, and some of the other countries with relatively favorable life expectancies were beginning to close the gap.

By the late 1960s and early 1970s, Cuba had become the country in the region with the highest life expectancy, followed closely by Costa Rica. Both these countries had surpassed Argentina, which by then had a life expectancy similar to those estimated for Panama, Paraguay, and Venezuela. Buenos Aires, however, was considerably ahead of Havana throughout the years, by ten years or more. The difference was still significant during the 1950s, but has probably narrowed down considerably, given the higher levels of life expectancy in Cuba. As in Cuba, in Argentina the capital city has always led the rest of the country in terms of life expectancy.

It is apparent, then, that the trend of declining mortality in Argentina was quite different from that observed in other Latin American countries. It was generally more similar to what Abdel Omran has described as the accelerated model (discussed in the Introduction to this study). But the Argentinean pattern also presents unique characteristics, since the country has been unable to sustain a continuous trend of declining mortality in recent years.

Cuba, and to a lesser extent Costa Rica, also differ from other countries in the region. Their experience only partially fits Omran's typology, since they appear to be intermediate cases, between the accelerated and the contemporary models. They began to experience mortality declines earlier than most other developing countries, and their secular trends of mortality decline were more gradual. At present they have reached life expectancy levels higher than the regional average, levels comparable to those observed in the industrialized nations.

Summary of the Mortality Trend from the
Nineteenth Century to the 1970s

The scanty data available on mortality in Cuba in the nineteenth century imply that mortality was very high and subject to violent fluctuations produced by epidemic diseases. By the turn of the century, a substantial decline in the levels of mortality became detectable as sanitary conditions improved following the Spanish-American War, and a new phase in the mortality transition became apparent as the wild, premodern fluctuations in the death rate disappeared. Mortality declined gradually during the first two decades of this century. The decline gained momentum in the 1920s, may have slowed down during the 1930s, and accelerated rapidly after the Second World War. That rapid decline appears to have continued through the 1960s. By 1970 Cuba had reached a life expectancy level comparable to that found in the developed countries. The present high level of life expectancy makes further large gains in life expectancy in Cuba doubtful.

Throughout the transition, the trends of mortality in Havana and in the rest of the country were roughly parallel, with Havana always in the lead. Except for Argentina and perhaps a few other developing nations in the Western Hemisphere for which data are not available, Cuba has led the region in mortality declines throughout the twentieth century. Important questions remain as to the causes of the mortality decline, however. It is the object of the next chapters to account for some of the causes.

Table 4
Estimated Life Expectancies for Selected Latin American Countries, Both Sexes Combined

Country	Estimated Life Expectancy (Years)							Most Recent Date[b]
	1900[a]	1910[a]	1920[a]	1930[a]	1940[a]	1950[a]	1960[a]	
Bolivia	25.5	28.5	31.6	34.7	38.8	43.1	—	47 (1975)
Brazil	29.4	30.6	32.0	34.0	36.7	43.0	55.5	60 (1974-75)
Chile	28.7	30.2	30.5	35.2	38.1	48.5	56.5	62 (1969-70)
Colombia	—	30.5	32.0	34.2	38.0	48.5	—	59 (1973)
Costa Rica	31.6	32.6	36.8	41.9	48.7	55.5	61.8	68 (1972-74)
Dominican Republic	—	—	—	26.1	34.0	43.7	52.2	55 (1965-70)
Ecuador	—	—	—	—	—	47.9	53.8	61 (1965-70)
El Salvador	—	—	—	28.7	37.5	47.2	56.0	55 (1969-72)
Guatemala	24.0	24.6	25.5	26.6	30.4	40.7	49.5	53 (1970-72)
Haiti	—	—	—	—	—	39.4	—	46 (1965-70)
Honduras	—	—	—	34.0	37.5	42.7	52.8	55 (1974)
Mexico	25.3	27.6	34.0	33.9	38.8	47.6	58.0	60 (1969-71)
Nicaragua	—	—	24.3	28.6	34.5	40.1	49.0	53 (1971)
Panama	—	—	—	35.9	42.4	50.2	61.5	65 (1969-71)
Paraguay	26.2	28.5	31.0	34.5	39.2	45.8	54.0	66 (1972)
Peru	—	—	—	—	36.5	39.9	48.5	55 (1970-75)
Venezuela	—	—	31.3	32.5	38.7	52.6	62.2	65 (1971)

Table 4—Continued

Country	Estimated Life Expectancy (Years)						
Argentina	1869-1895[c]	1895-1914[c]	1913-1915[c]	1946-1948[c]	1959-1961[c]	1969-1970[b]	
	32.9	40.0	48.5	61.1	66.4	66.0	
Buenos Aires	1894-1896[d]	1903-1905[d]	1908-1910[d]	1913-1915[d]	1935-1937[d]	1947[d]	1959-1961[d]
	40.9	47.7	46.9	48.6	59.4	65.2	70.7

Sources:

[a] Eduardo E. Arriaga, *New Life Tables for Latin American Populations in the Nineteenth and Twentieth Centuries*, Population Monograph Series, no. 3 (Berkeley and Los Angeles: University of California Press, 1968).

[b] Bureau of the Census, U.S. Department of Commerce, *World Population 1979: Recent Demographic Estimates for the Countries and Regions of the World*, ISP-WP-79 (Washington, D.C., 1980).

[c] Jorge L. Somoza, *La mortalidad en la Argentina entre 1869 y 1960* (Buenos Aires: Centro de Investigaciones Sociales, Instituto Torcuato di Tella and Centro Latinoamericano de Demografía, 1971), p. 26.

[d] Maria S. Muller, *La mortalidad en Buenos Aires entre 1855 y 1960* (Buenos Aires: Centro de Investigaciones Sociales, Instituto Torcuato di Tella and Centro Latinoamericano de Demografía, 1974), p. 19.

3. The Premodern Period and the Initial Mortality Decline

Mortality from Infectious Diseases in the Nineteenth Century

In nineteenth-century Cuba, the high level of mortality and its erratic variations from year to year reflected primarily the incidence of infectious diseases and their epidemic outbreaks. Only at the close of the century did this pattern change, as the frequency and severity of epidemics were reduced. For the first time, a gradual decline in mortality began.

During much of the nineteenth century, Cuba provided an ideal environment for epidemic diseases to take hold. By the 1820s, the island, which had stagnated economically for centuries, was well into what was to become one of its most rapid periods of economic expansion.[1] Most of the economic growth resulted from rising demand for Cuban sugar in the world markets. An inflow of free immigrants began partly in response to the booming economic conditions, and hundreds of thousands of slaves and indentured laborers from China were brought into the country to satisfy the rising demands for labor.[2]

Because of world-wide conditions in trade and travel prevalent at the time, and because of a disregard for proper sanitation, it is not surprising that the country provided an atmosphere in which epidemics could flare up. And flare up they did.[3] Cholera, dysentery, typhoid fever, yellow fever, and other diseases, singly and in conjunction, repeatedly took heavy tolls in lives.

Cholera was a frequent and dreaded visitor, and something to be expected, given the extensive international commerce conducted through Cuban ports. The approximate dates of cholera epidemics in Cuba correspond with dates of epidemics of the disease in other parts of the world at the time.[4] Violent cholera eruptions occurred in Havana in the early 1830s, during the 1850s, and late in the 1860s.[5] The epidemic of the 1830s was probably the most virulent ever recorded in the city: the Havana records indicate that in just fifty-four days, 8,465 persons fell victim to the disease in the Havana area alone; 435 succumbed on the single day of March 28, 1833. The 1850-1854 epidemic left 6,180 dead in Havana, and over 17,000 perished throughout the colony.[6]

The extent to which colonial mortality conditions in the major population enclaves—Havana in particular—and in the rural areas differed is difficult to establish. Historical records indicate that throughout the nineteenth century, mortality levels were high in the country's principal cities and that even the most basic sanitary standards were poorly implemented. As late as the close of the century, when the benefits that could be gained from sanitary measures had already been proved in cities in Europe and the United States, Spanish colonial authorities still lagged in following suit.[7]

The tendency of European migrants to concentrate in urban areas also contributed to heavy mortality in cities. The nonnatives were more susceptible to various diseases—especially yellow fever—than was the native-born population.[8]

The figures on numbers of deaths caused by cholera given by J. E. Le-Roy y Cassá, and other evidence, call into question, however, the assumption that Havana and other cities had significantly higher mortality than the rest of the country, at least during times of epidemics. During the nineteenth century, when the heavily settled areas of Cuba were concentrated in the central regions of the island, epidemics may have been as frequent and as destructive in those areas as in Havana. Cuban population enclaves, especially in the sugar regions, were located near a seaport or protected cove, where the bulky sugar could be easily loaded into ships. Epidemics could have spread easily to local populations through these ports. At the time, Cuba had practically no roads, and the railroads served very few regions. Furthermore, because the Spanish limited international trade, contraband and illicit trading were commonplace. It is very doubtful that smugglers or illegal slave-traders used the better-policed main ports, where either Spanish customs agents or British overseers of the ban on slave traffic were posted. In addition, even assuming that most slaves and indentured servants entered the country through Havana, where the main slave markets were located, they were rapidly distributed to the sugar plantations, and illegally smuggled slaves were likely to have bypassed major urban centers and found their way directly into rural areas.

If these observations are correct, the whole population of the colony was probably as exposed as the population of the City of Havana to epidemic diseases. Hugh Thomas has indicated that on the sugar plantations "epidemics were often very serious—in particular yellow fever and occasionally cholera."[9] During the 1833 cholera epidemic, the Spanish colonial governor estimated that some 55,000 slaves died over a two-month period, but he may have underestimated the number, since many of the slaves were not buried in the church cemeteries from which the estimates were taken, but rather in cemeteries belonging to the sugar mills.[10] That estimate, however, suggests that deaths among slaves in rural areas may have been very substantial during epidemics. Franklin W. Knight states that "the opinions expressed about slave mortality, as about everything else on the island, differed considerably. The only general consensus seemed to be that mortality rates were higher in the rural areas than in the towns, and highest of all on the sugar plantations."[11] Thus it would appear that high mortality of white immigrants in urban areas was more than counterbalanced by high mortality among the slave and laboring population in rural parts of the country.

Cause-of-death statistics for Havana during the 1880 to 1902 period (not available in such detail for other parts of the country) provide a quantified view of the conditions that prevailed in the city during the years immediately preceding the onset of the mortality decline. Table 5 lists Havana's annual crude death rates and cause-specific death rates for which data are available for this period. Figure 3 depicts salient features of the trends. Deaths attributed to yellow fever, smallpox, malaria, diphtheria, infantile tetanus, typhoid fever, and tuberculosis accounted for approximately one-third to one-half of all deaths recorded in the city in each year from 1880 to 1898, except in 1885 and 1886, when their share of the total dropped somewhat below one-third. It is apparent that the fluctuating incidence of these diseases accounted for most of the year-to-year variations in the overall levels of mortality during this period. If tuberculosis-related deaths are excluded, the predominance of these infectious diseases in the annual variations is accentuated, since heavy tuberculosis mortality was chronic in the city.

The incidence of all the infectious diseases fluctuated a great deal, but some fluctuated more than others. Smallpox, for example, exhibited the classic epidemic swings and reached in some years (1887, for instance) higher levels than tuberculosis.[12] Yellow fever, malaria, diphtheria, and, to a lesser extent, typhoid fever, exhibited patterns more like those of endemic diseases, that is, a fairly high level of incidence, aggravated from time to time by cyclical flare-ups. The trends for infantile tetanus and diphtheria differed from those of other infectious idiseases because they showed only moderate increases or reductions in their incidence as causes of death during the war years. A decline in fertility during the war years, or a reduction in the proportionate share of children in the population declined as soldiers and other adults temporarily settled in the city may partly explain these features of the trends for infantile tetanus and diphtheria.[13]

The death rate reached tremendously high levels between 1896 and 1898, well above the average levels of previous years. These levels were a direct result of the pathetic health and sanitary conditions that prevailed during the 1895-1898 War of Independence. The warring Cuban and Spanish armies set out systematically to destroy the economy of the country. The Spaniards took this course to deny the means of subsistence to the Cuban armies in the field, and the Cubans, to do away with the wealth that made the colony profitable to Spain. Sugar production dropped, from over 1,000,000 tons in 1894, to slightly more than 200,000 tons in 1897, and tobacco and banana exports, significant sources of income for certain segments of the population, were drastically curtailed.[14] By the end of the war, 90 percent of Cuba's livestock had been sacrificed.[15] The countryside was completely ravaged.

Already-poor sanitary standards in the cities deteriorated further as colonial authorities directed their attention to military activities. Epidemic outbreaks were more severe than ever, partly because the Spanish Army forced the rural population to concentrate in heavily garrisoned urban centers. Overcrowding and malnutrition led to the more facile spread and increased virulence of disease. Newly arrived Spanish soldiers fell victim to yellow fever, malaria, and other diseases to which they had not been exposed before. Food shortages were widespread and "desolation, starvation and chaos prevailed everywhere."[16]

The increase in the tuberculosis death rate was consistent with the influx of the rural population into urban centers, since crowding leads to greater contagion, and malnutrition tends to aggravate the consequences of the disease. Particularly remarkable was the increase in tuberculosis deaths in 1898. From April 21, when the United States declared war on Spain, to August 12, when an armistice was signed, the American navy blockaded Cuban ports, which resulted in a serious shortage of food and in conditions similar to those recorded in Havana in other cities. On January 1, 1899, Spain formally granted possession of Cuba to the United States, and the United States Army then took over the administration of the country.

The Initial Decline of Mortality, 1899-1902

The conditions that the American forces found in Cuba impelled them to take immediate and drastic measures in order to cope with the misery, famine, and disease that pervaded the country.[17] Table 5 and figure 3 display the results of those measures. By 1901 the level of mortality in the city had declined substantially, not only as a result of the end of the war (as famine- and war-related deaths stopped), but also as a result of a remarkable decline

Rate per
100,000 population

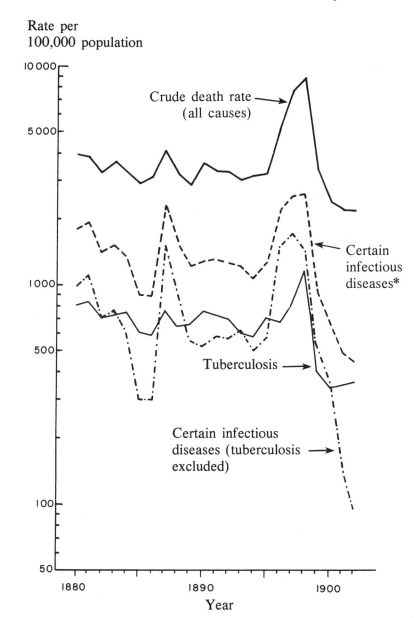

*Yellow fever, smallpox, malaria, diphtheria, infantile tetanus, typhoid fever, and tuberculosis.

Figure 3. Crude and Cause-Specific Death Rates for Certain Infectious Diseases, City of Havana

Table 5
Cause-Specific Death Rates for Certain Infectious Diseases, City of Havana
(Per 100,000 Inhabitants)

| Year | Disease | | | | | | | | Crude Death Rate (All Causes) |
	Yellow Fever (1)	Smallpox (2)	Malaria (3)	Diphtheria (4)	Infantile Tetanus (5)	Typhoid Fever (6)	Tuberculosis (7)	Total (1)-(7)	
1880	323.7	223.8	168.1	32.1	170.6	79.8	817.6	1815.7	3986.1
1881	243.2	354.0	114.3	38.6	190.0	161.5	842.0	1943.6	3894.9
1882	365.2	0.5	95.7	16.5	159.8	66.1	715.0	1418.8	3223.2
1883	425.0	2.5	91.6	26.0	155.2	77.1	736.4	1513.8	3674.9
1884	255.6	0.5	98.0	19.0	153.0	87.0	748.8	1361.9	3294.1
1885	82.4	0	50.5	16.0	98.9	57.5	619.2	924.5	2910.0
1886	83.4	0	67.4	11.0	94.4	55.4	592.7	904.3	3153.6
1887	265.4	825.2	134.2	68.3	167.1	87.8	761.8	2309.8	4171.6
1888	229.5	269.7	102.0	62.8	178.0	74.5	650.3	1566.8	3239.1
1889	146.1	3.4	109.9	49.7	165.4	85.8	666.4	1226.7	2856.1
1890	146.1	5.7	80.6	49.8	168.4	86.8	761.7	1299.1	3604.0
1891	166.1	70.4	94.7	36.4	149.3	71.8	729.3	1318.0	3382.4
1892	163.9	0	92.8	38.6	117.5	168.0	701.6	1282.4	3315.7
1893	224.2	3.6	108.5	66.4	127.4	94.0	606.6	1230.7	3026.9
1894	170.0	96.1	89.4	33.8	77.0	44.5	584.7	1095.5	3160.0

Table 5—*Continued*

Year	Disease							Total (1)-(7)	Crude Death Rate (All Causes)
	Yellow Fever (1)	Smallpox (2)	Malaria (3)	Diphtheria (4)	Infantile Tetanus (5)	Typhoid Fever (6)	Tuberculosis (7)		
1895	242.3	79.3	90.3	11.0	78.9	80.2	711.3	1293.3	3226.3
1896	553.4	433.4	194.2	8.2	100.2	210.2	681.2	2180.8	5077.5
1897	364.9	597.1	344.9	15.3	91.4	288.8	819.2	2521.6	7713.1
1898	57.0	70.4	799.3	9.6	72.5	423.3	1171.1	2603.2	8907.5
1899	42.6	1.6	375.5	16.1	38.0	57.8	405.3	936.9	3368.2
1900	124.5	0.8	138.2	6.0	55.8	36.2	341.8	703.3	2451.2
1901	7.0	0	59.0	9.8	50.0	32.4	351.8	510.1	2235.8
1902	0	0	29.3	9.5	25.9	33.1	361.2	459.0	2219.9

below the prewar levels of deaths due to infectious epidemic diseases. Over a two- or three-year span, the death rate in Havana dropped 30 percent below the prewar average-level, from around thirty deaths per thousand population or higher to the low twenties. This rapid and decisive decline in mortality is statistically recorded only for Havana, but sufficient written accounts exist to indicate that the decline was general throughout the country. The extensive sanitary reforms instituted by the American occupation forces reached the interior of the country, but later evidence clearly shows that the reforms were more effective in Havana.

The sanitary-reform movement, which had dramatically changed health conditions in Western Europe, North America, and other areas during the 1890s, provided a ready-made apparatus through which sweeping changes could rapidly be made. Effective programs were instituted to combat those diseases for which remedies were known. For instance, between July 1 and October 1, 1900, 50,342 persons were vaccinated against smallpox in the City of Havana alone (almost a quarter of the population of the city).[18] Reports from other regions of Cuba indicate that similar vaccination programs were carried out all over the country.[19]

The sanitation campaigns and reforms revolutionized the health standards of the country, particularly in the larger towns. The better-documented historical record for Havana illustrates how thorough these measures were.

During the year 1900, each house in the city was inspected three times, the result of each inspection being carefully recorded on a printed form in the office of the chief sanitary officer. Besides the work done by owners and tenants, under the direction of inspectors, more than half the houses were overhauled by the cleaning brigades of the sanitary department . . . . The Cleaning Department, the first six months of the year, cleaned 7,331 houses and removed 2,730½ carts of refuse . . . . Since the first of July, it has cleaned 7,637 houses and removed 3,323¾ carts of refuse.[20]

Among the many other measures instituted between 1899 and 1901 were burial regulations, a reorganization of the health-statistics service, quarantine regulations for international travelers, inspection of and regulations concerning the establishments where food was sold or prepared, and renewed attention to former plans for drainage, sewage, and street paving in the cities, and to the formulation of new plans.[21]

The crowning achievement of the military government was the program for eradication of yellow fever. The Yellow Fever Commission, acting on the theories of Carlos Finlay, conclusively proved that mosquitoes were the main vehicle by which this disease was transmitted to man.[22] The verification of Finlay's theory led to a vigorous campaign to destroy the breeding grounds of mosquitoes by draining swamps, spreading oil over stagnant waters, and using insecticides in places where known cases of yellow fever had been found (to destroy infected mosquitoes). In addition, yellow fever cases were isolated to prevent the spread of the disease. As table 5 makes evident, the campaign against yellow fever was a tremendous success, so much so that in 1902, not a single case was reported in Havana. The Havana data show that during the 1899-1902 period, malaria mortality also declined sharply, since the attack on the mosquito carriers of yellow fever also was extended to those that carried malaria.[23] However, malaria was to remain for many years a serious health problem in Cuba.

Figure 3 shows that the death rate from the group of "certain infectious diseases," with the exception of tuberculosis, was reduced in Havana from more than 1,400 per 100,000 in 1898, to 118 per 100,000 in 1902—that is, to approximately one-third of the lowest level recorded in any of the years between 1880 and 1898. Although we lack corresponding measures for the rest of the country, the evidence noted above implies that the sanitary reforms instituted between 1899 and 1902 had a significant effect on mortality from infectious diseases at least in urban centers, and probably also in rural areas.

The experience of Cuba in this period is one of the earliest examples of a major improvement in mortality brought about by the application in a less-developed country of disease-control technology imported from a more-developed country.[24] What was done in Cuba at this time appears to have been an important prerequisite for the continuing, more gradual decline of mortality during the next two decades. It also seems to explain why, by the early twentieth century, Cuba had attained life expectancy levels generally higher than the regional Latin American average (as discussed in Chapter 2). The decline beween 1898 and 1901 was achieved primarily by means of governmental decisions and expenditures, specifically in the areas of environmental sanitation and control of disease vectors.[25] Since the mortality decline occurred in such a short span of time, we can discard the possibility that other influences, such as economic improvements and better nutrition, had a major role.[26] The government responsible for instituting the measures leading to the mortality decline in this case was not that of the people whose health conditions improved, but a foreign government. This action on the part of the United States government was intended to protect the health of its own people as well as that of the people of Cuba.

4. The Context of the Mortality Decline in the First Half of the Twentieth Century

Before I begin my analysis of the factors that may have been involved in the mortality decline in Cuba during the 1901-1953 period, I shall describe some of the political, economic, and social factors that may have contributed to the decline. First I shall review political events that appear to have been overwhelmingly significant in the Cuban case, particularly during the first decades of the century. Then I shall attempt to assess the way in which the Cuban economy grew or stagnated during these years. Finally, I shall assess the secular development of certain variables that, although not fully dependent on economic growth per se, may be closely associated with it. After having set the stage by describing some of the more salient socioeconomic characteristics of the country, I shall analyze the determinants of the mortality decline by considering how these factors and advances in medical knowledge may have affected the secular trends of cause-specific mortality.

Political Factors

After nearly four years of military occupation, Cuba gained its independence from the United States in 1902. However, this independence was constrained by a number of provisions in an amendment the United States forced into the Cuban constitution to regulate future relations between the two nations (the Platt Amendment). The amendment granted the United States government the right to intervene in Cuban affairs if certain conditions were not met by the national government. Of particular interest to the present study is the paragraph of the amendment that reads as follows:

That the government of Cuba will execute, and, as far as necessary, extend, the plans already devised or other plans to be mutually agreed upon, for the sanitation of the cities of the island, to the end that a recurrence of epidemic and infectious diseases may be prevented, thereby assuring protection to the people and commerce of Cuba, as well as to the commerce of the southern ports of the United States and the people residing therein.

This provision probably had a profound influence on the subsequent development of public health in Cuba, inasmuch as it obliged the Cuban government to maintain closer surveillance over the country's sanitary conditions than that maintained by the governments of other countries at similar levels of socioeconomic development early in this century. The literature of the time indicates that the government paid considerable attention to the preservation or improvement of public health standards within the limits imposed by the resources of the country, and to how the state of public health in Cuba was viewed in the United States.[1]

Other provisions of the Platt Amendment assured foreign capitalists safe and profitable investments in Cuba, because the American government maintained close supervision over Cuban political affairs and could intervene if necessary to protect United States interests. The first three decades of the century saw an unprecedented amount of foreign investment.[2] The result was a rapid expansion of the national economy, which may have contributed significantly to the decline of mortality. The growth of the economy permitted the expansion of infrastructural and sanitary facilities, raised national income levels, and contributed to improvements in nutrition and education, all factors favorable to a decline in mortality.

During a second United States administration of the country (1906-1909), the first nationwide health ministry in the world was established. Through this ministry the central government funded a public health apparatus in each of the country's municipalities.[3] Before 1907, sanitation efforts outside of the major urban centers had not been very successful, primarily because they were hampered by lack of funds and technical support. The reorganization of the public health system resulted directly in the extension to all parts of the country of at least rudimentary resources to improve sanitation and the means by which rapid action could be taken to curtail the spread of infectious diseases if outbreaks occurred. For example, local sanitation authorities reported daily to the national ministry on the prevalence of morbidity and mortality in their districts. Whenever alarming reports were received from local areas, medical teams and supplies were to be dispatched from Havana to investigate and correct the conditions. Although it would be credulous to assume that the system worked as originally envisioned—a vast amount of data for later years speaks to the contrary—it did contribute to health improvements throughout the country over the years.

The Platt Amendment was abrogated during the early 1930s, yet the influence of the United States on Cuban affairs remained overwhelming until the time of the socialist revolution. Medical advances occurring in the United States rapidly found their way into Cuba, and, at times, American foundations provided resources for the study and amelioration of some of Cuba's health problems. The politics of the country remained under American tutelage, and the economy remained highly vulnerable to forces beyond the nation's control.

Economic Factors

The Cuban economy during the first half of this century was heavily dependent on international demand for its agricultural commodities, especially sugar. The economy's reliance on sugar ranged from 70 to 90 percent of total Cuban exports over the period.[4] It has been estimated that in 1945 and 1947, 24 and 37 percent, respectively, of the total national income originated in the combined output of the milling and marketing of sugar;[5] and it is certain that in earlier years sugar accounted for a much higher share of national income.

This extreme dependency on sugar had both positive and negative effects on the economic development of the country. On the one hand, during the early decades of the century, it allowed Cuba to attain a relatively high degree of prosperity.[6] On the other, it created conditions that made sustained economic growth difficult later, since fluctuations in the international demand for sugar, together with the wide oscillations of sugar prices, resulted in serious impediments to continuous growth. The country was particularly vulnerable to changes in its foreign-trade position, partly because of structural rigidities and partly because of overspecialization.

As a result of the erratic fluctuations in prices of and demand for sugar in the world markets, investors in Cuba placed more faith in short-term gains from rising sugar demand and prices than in the lower rates of return they could expect from investments in other areas of the economy. High liquidity as a buffer against cyclical fluctuations dominated the thinking of Cuban capitalists. Henry Wallich referred to this lack of economic aggressiveness as the "sugar mentality," and attributed to it much of the economic stagnation in the country during the second quarter of the century.[7] The World Bank noted that Cubans had a "gambling spirit in economics," which made them see long-term investments as undesirable when quick, high profits could be made as a result of erratic upturns in the world demand for sugar.[8]

The unfavorable position of the country as an exporter of raw materials and as an importer of manufactured goods was a major cause of stagnation in the Cuban economy. The hypothesis of deterioration in terms of trade, postulated by Raúl Prebisch and other economists affiliated with the United Nations' Economic Commission for Latin America, maintains that this position was one of the principal reasons why the region failed to develop.

Many students of Cuban affairs have stated that political factors (that is, imperialism) contributed a great deal to the economic stagnation of the country. In many respects American interests dominated the national economy, and these interests did not always correspond with those of Cuba.[9] Bilateral trade arrangements, for example, had negative consequences for the development of native industries, as did Cuba's lack of raw materials, the limited size of its internal markets, and other factors.

Figure 4 assesses the secular trend of growth of the Cuban economy, as well as its instability, from 1903 to 1948 (in actual and real dollars, adjusted to the level of prices in 1926). The per capita income series was estimated by Julián Alienes y Urosa of the National Bank of Cuba.[10] The World Bank study cited earlier concluded that this series "may be accepted with considerable confidence as an indication of the relative magnitudes involved,"[11] but indicated that the "United States price data used to deflate the Cuban income series produce misleading results for the two war periods."[12] The chart indicates vigorous growth of per capita income during the first quarter of the century, followed by a period of decline or stagnation that lasted from shortly before the onset of the Great Depression to World War II. It is particularly striking that the per capita estimates (in real dollars) during the late 1940s are lower than those of the 1910 to 1925 period. The severe deterioration of the national economy during the 1930s is quite evident, as are the oscillations in per capita income in periods of both prosperity and depression.

Figure 5 assesses the extent to which the Cuban economy depended on exports. Living conditions were particularly dependent on the value of exports, since Cuba, overemphasizing the development of the sugar industry, neglected the development of other areas of the economy to the point where, although primarily an agricultural country, it depended heavily on the importation of agricultural goods for its food supply. The data in figure 5 show how dependent Cuban national income levels were on exports, and hence, how dependent the import levels were on export levels. When foreign exchange was scarce, food imports declined dramatically, as was the case during the depression of the 1930s.

Other noteworthy aspects of the Cuban economy were the unequal income distribution,[13] the almost total absence of subsistence agriculture,

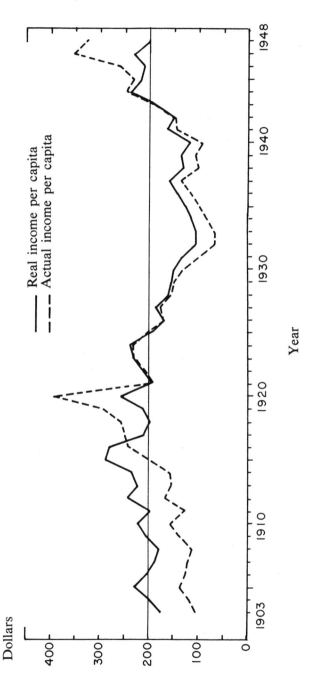

Figure 4. Cuban Per Capita Income in Actual and Real Dollars

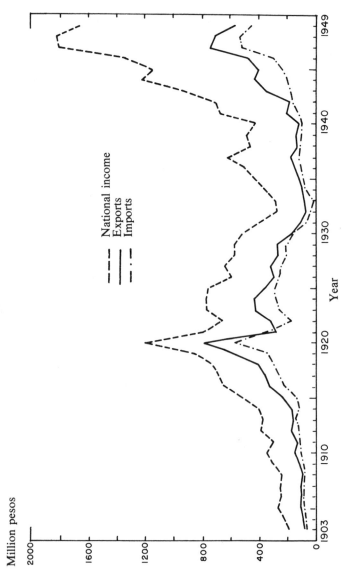

Figure 5. Cuban National Income, Exports, and Imports

Source: Julián Alienes y Urosa, *Características fundamentales de la economía cubana* (Havana: Banco Nacional de Cuba, 1950), p. 52; and International Bank for Reconstruction and Development (World Bank), *Report on Cuba* (Baltimore, Md.: Johns Hopkins University Press, 1951), p. 725.

and the highly seasonal character of economic activities. Productive activities revolved about the few months during which the sugarcane was harvested, and the remainder of the year was characterized by a lull described in Cuba as *el tiempo muerto* ("the dead season").

The heavy capitalization of the sugar industry led to a high degree of concentration of land in large holdings (latifundia). This, together with other historical and economic developments, minimized opportunities for subsistence agriculture. The more economically disadvantaged segment of the population got only marginal benefits in times of prosperity and suffered disproportionally in times of economic adversity.

Housing Conditions

If we compare the data on water supplies and means of sewage disposal provided in the censuses of 1899 and 1953, we can investigate to some extent the degree to which housing conditions improved in Cuba. These data are shown in tables 6 and 7. In both cases I have considered urban and rural differences for the country as a whole, as well as for the Province of Havana. Comparability is especially impaired by the differences in the census definitions of "urban localities." In the 1899 census the urban data refer only to the major cities and towns; in 1953, places with more than 150 inhabitants and having certain services were considered urban.

In general, the data show that percentages changed significantly from 1899 to 1953, and large qualitative changes surely occurred, particularly in the urban areas. The percentage of urban dwellings with toilet facilities increased greatly, and significantly more in the Havana area than elsewhere. The relative distribution of waste-disposal facilities in the rural areas of the country changed only slightly. The data for the Province of Havana, as we may have expected, do show some improvements, although the precise extent is difficult to interpret, since the definition of the urban component is different for the two dates.

The information regarding the percentage distribution by type of water supply (table 7) is somewhat baffling, since it appears that in the rural areas the percentage distribution actually deteriorated. The country as a whole, though, seems to have improved considerably, because the percentage of dwellings receiving water from aqueducts more than doubled over the period.[14] Differences in the definition of urban and rural areas, as well as many other variables, may affect these comparisons. Yet this evidence, with some additional data from the 1953 census, suggest that over the fifty-year span the improvements in housing were concentrated almost exclusively in urban areas.

Table 6
Distribution of Dwellings by Type of Human-Waste Disposal Facility
(Percentages)

	Facility Type				
	Toilet[a]	Privy[a]	None	Not Specified	Total
Cuba					
All areas					
1899	5.0	42.0	49.0	4.0	100.0
1953	42.0	35.0	23.0	—	100.0
Urban areas					
1899[b]	3.0	85.0	9.0	3.0	100.0
1953	62.0	33.0	5.0	—	100.0
Rural areas					
1899	—	32.0	65.0	3.0	100.0
1953	8.0	38.0	54.0	—	100.0
Province of Havana					
All areas					
1899	21.0	51.0	21.0	7.0	100.0
1953	81.0	13.0	6.0	—	100.0
Urban areas					
1899[c]	48.0	43.0	3.0	6.0	100.0
1953	86.0	12.0	2.0	—	100.0
Rural areas					
1899[d]	—	57.0	35.0	8.0	100.0
1953	16.0	27.0	57.0	—	100.0

Sources: United States War Department, *Census of Cuba, 1899*, pp. 176-178, 520; República de Cuba, *Censo de 1953*, pp. 209, 211, 213.

[a] The labels "toilet" and "privy" are assumed to correspond to those given in the 1899 census as *inodoro* and *pozo*, respectively. In that census volume it was noted that "the *inodoro* includes every receptacle for excreta in which an effort is made to destroy or decrease the foul odors arising therefrom, usually by the addition of such substances as lime, dry clay, or ashes. The *pozo* includes all other forms of closet. The modern form of closet flushed by water from a system of pipes, called *escusado inglés*, is very unusual in Havana, and unknown elsewhere in Cuba" (United States War Department, *Census of Cuba*, pp. 177-178, n. 1).

For 1953, under the label "toilet," the following categories were grouped: *inodoro interior, uso exclusivo; inodoro exterior, uso exclusivo;* and *inodoro exterior, uso varias.* Under "privy," the following categories were included: *letrina interior, uso exclusivo; letrina exterior, uso exclusivo;* and *letrina exterior, uso varias.*

[b] Does not include the City of Havana.

[c] City of Havana only.

[d] All of the province except the City of Havana.

Note: A dash signifies an unspecified category in that census.

Table 7
Distribution of Dwellings by Type of Water-Supply System
(Percentages)

			System Type		
	Aqueduct[a]	Cistern	Stream and Well	Not Specified	Total
Cuba					
All areas					
1899	16.0	46.0	35.0	3.0	100.0
1953	35.0	22.0	43.0	—	100.0
Urban areas					
1899	53.0	23.0	17.0	7.0	100.0
1953	55.0	27.0	18.0	—	100.0
Rural areas					
1899	2.0	54.0	42.0	2.0	100.0
1953	2.0	13.0	85.0	—	100.0
Province of Havana					
All areas					
1899	38.0	47.0	7.0	8.0	100.0
1953	65.0	25.0	10.0	—	100.0
Urban areas					
1899[b]	82.0	4.0	2.0	12.0	100.0
1953	70.0	25.0	5.0	—	100.0
Rural areas					
1899[c]	5.0	79.0	12.0	4.0	100.0
1953	7.0	19.0	74.0	—	100.0

Sources: United States War Department, *Census of Cuba. 1899*, pp. 171-174 and 514-515; República de Cuba, *Censo de 1953*, pp. 209, 211, and 213.

[a] The terms used at the headings of the columns are those that appear in the census volume for 1899. The corresponding percentages for 1953 have been derived from the following labels in the 1953 census tables: aqueduct (*agua de acueducto, interior*); cistern (*agua de aljibe interior, agua por tubería externa*); stream and well (*agua de río, pozo, o manantial*).

[b] City of Havana only.

[c] All of the province except the City of Havana.

Note: A dash signifies an unspecified category in that census.

The 1953 census reported that in rural Cuba, where 43 percent of the population lived, 66.2 percent of the dwellings had dirt floors, as opposed to no less than 6.4 percent in the urban areas.[15] Just as revealing is the fact that in 1953, in rural Cuba 75.4 percent of the dwellings had been built either of palm-trunk boards or of palm bark with a thatched roof of palm leaves. In urban areas as a whole, dwellings of this type constituted only 9.7 percent of the total, and in the urban areas of the Province of Havana, only 3.0 percent.[16]

In conclusion, although conditions in the rural areas hardly changed during this period, the housing conditions of the total population improved, partly because of the increase in urbanization. These improvements undoubtedly had a beneficial effect on the health standards of the population.

Water Supply Sources and Sewerage Systems

Safe water supplies and sewerage systems are intimately associated with advances in sanitary conditions. However, as the previous section suggested, important sanitary improvements with regard to water and sewerage can have taken place only in the urban areas, since the situation in rural Cuba in 1953 was still rather primitive.

As early as June 1903, the national government appropriated money for construction of the aqueducts for the provincial capitals of Camagüey and Santiago de Cuba, as well as for an extension of the water-supply system of Havana (probably the only Cuban city with fairly adequate facilities at that time).[17] Somewhat later considerable other expenditures were made to improve, repair, and extend the water-supply systems of cities all over the country.[18] Between 1909 and 1913, 9,883,109 pesos were spent in the development and expansion of the sewerage system of the City of Havana— a fairly sizable part of the national budgets during those years.[19]

The 1943 census provided data that can be used for gross estimates of the extent to which the urban population of Cuba was served by aqueducts. It was stated in this census volume that 112 aqueducts were in operation in the country (35 of them under state or municipal control, the rest in private hands, or less than 1 for each of the 126 Cuban municipalities). Of the total number of aqueducts, 45, or about 40 percent, attempted to purify the water by some chemical means.[20] It was noted that only 2 of the aqueducts had been constructed between 1932 and 1943, which indicates that most of the progress in the area of water supply occurred during the years of Cuba's economic expansion and reflects on the serious economic circumstances which the country underwent during the 1930s.[21]

The aqueducts were far from being equally distributed throughout the country, and even though the sewerage network was unevenly extended to cover some of the major towns, it was insufficient, since the country was rapidly urbanizing and experiencing high population growth. The fact that the city of Santiago de Cuba, the country's second largest, was estimated to have under normal conditions only two-thirds of the water needed for a city of that size suggests that the water and sewerage systems were highly inadequate throughout the country. Further, many visitors and residents of that city suffered from gastrointestinal disturbances because the water was notoriously impure and the aqueduct lacked a water-treatment plant.[22]

In short, the water and sewerage systems were generally poorly developed in Cuba. Although some progress did occur over time, it was confined mainly to urban areas, and, as the evidence from Santiago de Cuba indicates, the improvements were not as substantial as they could have been, compared to what conditions had been in the early part of the century. In this area, as in many others, Havana was in a class by itself.

Literacy

The evidence suggests that increased literacy may have played a substantial role in the country's mortality decline. At various times and to different extents, the government conducted campaigns to educate the public in the means to combat many diseases. These efforts included distribution of free pamphlets that dealt with the nature, cure, and prevention of certain diseases, mainly of the infectious or contagious types.

Table 8 shows that the literacy of the Cuban population over ten years of age improved greatly during the first three decades of this century. After 1931 only minor improvements were recorded, and between 1943 and 1953, the trend

Table 8
Literacy of the Population over Ten Years of Age

Census Year	% Literate
1899[a]	43.2
1907	56.6
1919	61.6
1931	71.7
1943	77.9
1953	76.4

Source: Cuban censuses.

[a] Includes 2.7 percent who stated that they could read, only.

reversed. Higher literacy levels prevailed in the urban areas and in the Province of Havana than elsewhere in the country. In 1953, for example, over 90 percent of the province's population over ten years of age could read and write.

The importance of literacy as a factor in the mortality decline was probably greatest in the years before the chemical revolution began (after the Second World War, for the most part). By that time mass governmental efforts made possible the control of many diseases which until then had been fought mainly through individual initiative.

Rural-Urban Population Shifts

Between 1899 and 1953 the proportion of Cuba's population living in areas classified as urban rose from 47 to 57 percent (see table 9), but we cannot assess with certainty the influence of this increase on the country's mortality trend. Whereas the life tables for Havana and Cuba suggest that mortality was lower in Havana than in the country as a whole throughout the first half of the twentieth century, no comparable data are available to test whether mortality was lower in the other urban areas than in the rural parts of the country. Although the health advantages generally found in urban areas (for example, concentration of health facilities, superior housing, better educational facilities) may have made for lower mortality in towns and small cities, the detrimental effects on health of high population-density and problems in the provision of adequate urban sanitation services, water supplies, and sewerage systems may have outweighed these advantages. Since sanitary facilities in Cuban towns and cities other than Havana were seldom adequate, it is unlikely that their mortality levels were as low as Havana's.

Table 9
Percentage of Cuba's Total Population Residing in Urban Areas,
in Municipality of Havana, and in Metropolitan Havana

Census Year	% in All Urban Areas	% in Municipality of Havana	% in Metropolitan Havana
1899	47.1	16.1	—
1907	43.9	14.8	18.3
1919	44.7	12.6	16.5
1931	51.4	13.7	18.5
1943	54.6	14.2	20.0
1953	57.0	13.5	21.3

Source: Cuban censuses.

Note: Dash signifies that data were not available.

Nevertheless, Havana continued to have lower mortality than the rest of the country while a somewhat larger proportional share of the total population of Cuba resided in metropolitan Havana in 1953 than in the early years of the century.[23] Hence, we may assume that the increasing concentration of the country's population in Havana contributed somewhat to the decline of mortality in the country as a whole.

Nutrition

The lack of a secular series on caloric consumption per head makes the extent to which nutritional levels changed in Cuba over time difficult to assess. The available information appears to show that, in general, the nutritional levels of the Cuban population were not exceptionally inadequate. Although we should not expect the Cuban level to have matched those in the more developed countries, they appear to have been superior to those found in most developing countries: "In the mid-1950s Cubans seem to have had enough to eat in that their daily per capita calorie intake (2,740 calories) was higher than their estimated requirement (2,460). The occasional general or local famines that plague some Latin American countries were unknown, and most Cubans ate two meals a day."[24] However, the dietary habits of the population were not well suited to proper nutrition, since the typical Cuban—even in the higher-income groups—preferred a diet high in carbohydrates.[25]

The most comprehensive study ever made of the nutritional status of the Cuban population, conducted by Norman Jolliffe and associates, reviews earlier investigations of nutritional conditions in the country.[26] Jolliffe noted that nutritional deficiencies in the Cuban diet had existed for over one hundred years, as witnessed by infantile protein malnutrition and avitaminosis (vitamin deficiency). He concluded that the Cuban diet was similar to that of the United States in amount of ascorbic acid, carbohydrates, and iron, but deficient in calcium, vitamin A, and riboflavin. However, anemia and low hemoglobin were not major problems among school-age children in Cuba. Jolliffe found that the two principal sources of calories in the average Cuban diet were rice, which accounted for 22.2 percent of the total calorie intake, and sugar, which provided 17.5 percent. These findings led the authors to recommend vitamin enrichment of the staple food, rice, as an extremely valuable contribution to public health.[27] A similar conclusion had been reached earlier by the World Bank.[28] Nutritional levels among poor rural workers were likely to be worse than among the better-off population of the cities, a conclusion supported by some limited evidence.[29]

Because rice was such an important element in the average diet, we can make gross estimates of changes in the nutritional intake of the population by using the per capita consumption of rice as a proxy. During the first four decades of this century, when most of the rice consumed in the country was imported, authorities maintained a complete record of the quantities bought abroad. When it began to be produced locally in important amounts, production statistics were kept. Hence, it is possible to estimate an annual series of per capita consumption of rice, from 1902 to 1956.[30] In order to minimize the year-to-year variability in the series likely to have been produced by price fluctuations, changes in the supplies of foreign exchange, and inventory adjustments, I have smoothed the series by computing five-year moving averages. The resulting series of per capita rice consumption is shown graphically in figure 6.

As the figure indicates, the consumption of rice on a per capita basis was very high in Cuba, about fifty kilograms a year. It is striking that the per capita consumption declined significantly after having achieved fairly high levels during the first quarter of the century. The earlier high consumption levels were not attained again until the late 1940s and early 1950s. These results are compatible with the per capita income trends described earlier and are also consistent with the observation that the levels of imports were very much dependent on the volume of exports. The rice consumption series suggests substantial declines in the calorie-consumption levels of the Cuban population during the years of economic crisis and, furthermore, appears to parallel the trends in life expectancy gains.

Medical Facilities

The number of physicians in proportion to population is one indicator of the extent to which a country's population has access to health care. Even under conditions in which medical intervention per se may not have contributed significantly to a decline in mortality, we can expect that physicians had an important role in the dissemination of knowledge about public health and sanitation to the general population.

Data on population per physician, presented in table 10 for Cuba, the Province of Havana, and the City of Havana, suggest that in this regard the country was relatively well off. The unsteady increase in the ratio (which implies deterioration in availability of medical care) during the first third of the century probably resulted from the arrival of thousands of immigrants, most of whom had low skill levels. The noticeable deterioration in 1931 may have been influenced further by the fact that political instability caused the closing of the national university for a number of years around that time. By 1953 the ratio of population to physicians had dropped to a level that was probably one of the most favorable in the developing world.

We may infer large regional disparities in the availability of physicians from

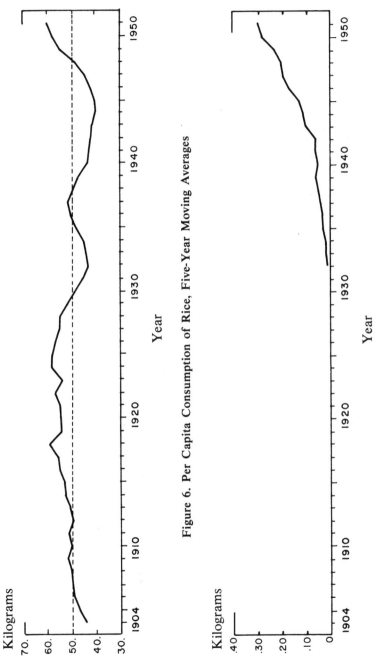

Figure 6. Per Capita Consumption of Rice, Five-Year Moving Averages

Figure 7. Per Capita Consumption of Insecticides, Five-Year Moving Averages

Table 10
Population per Physician

Census Year	Population per Physician		
	Cuba	Province of Havana	City of Havana
1899	1,286	649	488
1907	1,648	804	589
1919	1,631	691	531
1931	1,958	928	630
1943	1,846	763	—
1953	940	—	—

Source: Censuses of Cuba.

Note: A dash signifies data not available.

the table. Physicians were highly concentrated in the Havana area and, to a lesser extent, in other urban areas, particularly the provincial capitals. In some of the rural areas, the shortage of doctors was severe throughout the period.[31] As might be expected, the better doctors and superior medical facilities were concentrated in the national capital, but even outside of the major urban centers, some minimal, if largely inadequate, medical attention was provided. A study conducted by the Foreign Policy Association in the early 1930s disclosed that each municipality employed at least one physician to provide medical attention to the poor, a finding consistent with the reorganization of the national health system in 1907. Most of these medical services were provided on a dispensary plan, with few home visits by physicians. Also, an "island-wide system of public hospitals" was financed by the state,[32] although hospital facilities were largely concentrated in major cities.[33]

A peculiar institution that flourished in Cuba and exerted a favorable influence on the health conditions of a substantial segment of the population was the mutualist health association. These societies were first established during the late nineteenth century to serve the medical needs of poor Spanish immigrants, but were eventually expanded to provide services to a wider cross section of the population. For a modest fee they provided access to a wide range of medical services and to the use of hospital facilities, at no extra cost. It was estimated that in metropolitan Havana in 1914, close to 25 percent of the population were members of these associations.[34] By 1927 this membership had increased to nearly half of the population of metropolitan Havana.[35]

Although they were concentrated in Havana, many of those associations had local branches in other areas of the country, and members from those areas were entitled to utilize the centrally located facilities in Havana under the same conditions as the local members. Local mutual associations could also be found in some of the country's major cities.[36] These societies thrived for many years and continued to expand until a few years after the socialist revolution in the late 1950s.

The important point is that these associations provided medical services not dependent on governmental revenues, and the government was able to provide at least limited medical services to the segment of the population unable to pay the fees required to join the mutual associations.[37] Consequently, the mutual associations provided services that the government alone could not have given—ranging from the purely medical to the dissemination of public-health information. In sum, public and private medical facilities appear to have been adequate in urban centers of the country, especially in Havana, but in rural areas the situation was very different, since both medical facilities and personnel were generally in short supply.

Technological Factors

Among the factors that certainly influenced the Cuban mortality decline were the availability of sulfonamides after the mid-1930s and of antibiotics after World War II, and the appearance of residual insecticides in 1945. An examination of the Cuban mortality records supports the assumption that the modern drugs were widely used almost from the time they first began to be used by civilian populations in developed countries. The carefully kept statistics on imports provide information about the probable impact of the residual insecticides on Cuban mortality.[38]

A series on the amount of insecticides imported yearly into Cuba, on a per capita basis, is shown graphically in figure 7. The upturn in the curve is consistent with the fully described use of DDT to destroy the malaria-carrying mosquitoes in Ceylon, British Guiana, and other countries. Malaria was endemic in certain areas of Cuba, as will be shown later, and health authorities had paid it special attention during the 1930s.

5. The Mortality Decline in Havana, 1901-1953

A structural analysis of trends of death rates in terms of age groups and causes of death is helpful for an insight into determinants of the mortality decline. As mortality declines, marked changes in the incidence of death by age and cause occur. These changes and the time at which they take place serve as sensitive indicators of the causative forces inducing mortality declines and help to interpret the well-being of a society. The overall characteristics of these structural shifts, except for minor deviations, appear to be common to all societies (see Chapter 1). This chapter investigates how closely the Cuban mortality decline fits the general pattern of structural changes and tries to identify the periods at which those changes occurred. The Cuban statistics furnish a firmer basis for an analysis of the trends in the City of Havana during the first half of the twentieth century than is available for the rest of the country.

Age Groups

Table 11 presents the age pattern of declining mortality in Havana in terms of age-sex-specific death rates (that is, number of deaths per year of a given age and sex per one thousand of the city's population in corresponding age-sex groups) in the census years from 1901 to 1953. Throughout this period, mortality declined in all age groups of both sexes, except for some apparent increases in certain groups between 1901 and 1907. The significance of the apparent changes between 1901 and 1907 is uncertain because the reliability of the measures for 1901 is relatively low. Throughout the half-century period, the decline of the rates was more pronounced in age groups under forty-five years than in older groups, and the rates recorded for females decreased more than those for males.[1]

Table 11
Annual Death Rates per 1,000 Population,
by Sex and Age, City of Havana

Age Group	Census Year					
Males	1901	1907	1919	1931	1943	1953
Less than 1	252.9	204.6	130.9	94.4	82.3	59.2
1-4	25.1	24.6	20.4	11.8	10.7	3.7
5-14	4.0	4.9	4.1	2.7	2.4	1.4
15-24	9.8	8.1	10.9	5.5	4.5	2.2
25-44	16.3	13.6	17.7	9.8	8.1	4.2
45-64	43.2	40.3	48.9	33.8	28.3	22.0
65-74	117.1	114.4	121.2	104.7	80.0	69.9
75 and over	275.3	251.2	236.2	181.8	161.1	156.4
Females						
Less than 1	211.5	173.7	109.7	72.3	72.0	41.0
1-4	21.4	24.7	19.6	11.2	10.3	3.4
5-14	4.2	5.4	3.8	2.1	2.2	1.0
15-24	9.7	9.3	9.1	6.0	5.0	1.9
25-44	15.6	15.0	14.6	7.5	6.3	2.8
45-64	24.6	28.3	28.6	20.7	17.8	11.8
65-74	63.3	86.2	79.0	58.8	45.1	39.6
75 and over	128.9	203.0	192.9	152.7	127.4	113.5

Source: Cuban censuses and vital statistics.

Women, with a few exceptions, had consistently lower age-specific death rates than men. Across all age groups, the largest declines took place during the periods 1919-1931 and 1943-1953.

As Thomas McKeown and associates have noted, "The contribution of any age group [to the mortality decline in the whole population] is somewhat complex, being determined by the number of individuals in the group, the level of mortality and the rate of decline of mortality—all within the age group."[2] We can estimate the contribution of each age group to the decline of the overall death rate by calculating how many lives would have been saved in the population at the earliest date, had the terminal age-specific mortality rates been in effect.[3] Table 12 shows the results of those calculations for the periods 1901-1953 and 1907-1953 (since the 1901 rates are less reliable). In both cases, the age group that contributed most to the decline in the death rate is that of infants under one year of age

Table 12
Age Group Contribution to Total Decline in Death Rate,
Both Sexes Combined, City of Havana
(Percentages)

Age Group	1901-1953	1907-1953
Less than 1	29.5	24.3
1-4	7.9	12.2
5-14	3.8	4.3
15-24	11.2	10.6
25-44	27.4	24.1
45-64	14.2	14.2
65-74	3.8	5.4
75 and over	2.2	4.9
All ages	100.0	100.0

Source: Cuban censuses and vital statistics.

(especially for the estimates for 1901-1953), which is consistent with other evidence suggesting that infant mortality declined very rapidly between 1901 and 1907. Considering either period, we can attribute over 36 percent of the total decline in the death rate to the decrease in mortality of children under five years of age.

The very large savings of lives at ages fifteen to sixty-four, and more particularly at ages twenty-five to forty-four, are directly related to the large percentages of the total population of the city in those age groups (see table 13). When considering the data in tables 12 and 13, it becomes evident that the contribution of the age groups under five years of age was quite out of proportion to their share of the population. Although they accounted for only about 10 percent of the city's population, they contributed over 30 percent of the total decline in the death rate. This finding and the others reviewed above agree with the age patterns of mortality decline in other parts of the world. Life-table mortality rates ($_nq_x$) available for Havana and Cuba (Appendix 4) also indicate that Cuba's pattern of mortality decline by age is consistent with that observed elsewhere.

Causes of Death

I obtained a secular series of cause-of-death statistics for the City of Havana that consists of eleven major groupings that are mutually exclusive

Table 13
Age Distribution of Population, Both Sexes Combined,
City of Havana
(Percentages)

Age Group	Census Year					
	1901	1907	1919	1931	1943	1953
Less than 1	2.4	2.6	2.8	2.0	1.6	1.6
1-4	6.2	8.6	8.0	6.9	5.8	6.2
5-14	20.2	16.1	19.0	17.3	15.4	14.8
15-24	22.1	24.1	20.1	20.4	18.6	16.9
25-44	33.7	33.8	33.9	35.0	35.3	34.2
45-64	12.8	12.3	13.3	15.0	18.5	20.4
65-74	1.7	1.8	1.9	2.2	3.3	4.2
75 and over	0.7	0.8	0.9	1.0	1.3	1.7
All ages	100.0	100.0	100.0	100.0	100.0	100.0

Source: Cuban censuses.

and that include all registered deaths.[4] Within the eleven major groups, I was able to isolate fourteen specific causes or groups of causes of death extracted from the International List of Causes of Death, which permits a more detailed analysis, although in a few instances, the comparability is not perfect. In the text and the tables that follow, I will consider first the mutually exclusive causes, followed by the causes selected within the major groupings.[5]

Table 14 presents age-sex-standardized death rates specific for each cause-group or cause for Havana at six census dates. I computed them by standardizing the rates to the age-sex population structure in 1943, per 100,000 population. I corrected the population data for underenumeration of children under one year of age.

Table 15 shows the percentage contributions of each cause-group or cause to the mortality decline from 1901 to 1953, and for 1907 to 1953, for both sexes combined and by sex.[6] Respiratory tuberculosis appears as one of the greatest contributors to the mortality decline—especially for females. Respiratory and nonrespiratory tuberculosis accounted for nearly 25 percent of the mortality decline in the City of Havana. The other infectious and parasitic diseases contributed approximately 15 percent of the total decline, and benign and malignant tumors showed significant increases. Although it is almost certain that the mortality from benign and malignant tumors increased, it is sensible to believe that the increases resulted partially from the transference of cause of death from other cause groups, as diagnostic procedures improved.

Cardiovascular diseases were also responsible for a large share of the mortality decline. Samuel Preston and Verne Nelson, using data for many countries, found similar results in their analysis of changes in the cause-structure of mortality and held that, since many cardiovascular diseases are infectious, the decline of mortality from these should have been similar to that of other infectious diseases.[7]

The percentage declines from diarrhea, gastritis, and enteritis were substantially different between the estimates for 1901-1953 and 1907-1953. As stated earlier, this difference may reflect a great improvement between 1901 and 1907 in the survival rates of infants. This cause-group was among the major contributors to the mortality decline in the city.

The other major groupings did not seem to differ significantly between the two periods, with the exception of both diseases of infancy and accidents and violence. The latter cause-group was likely to be subject to more random variability, whereas the former may have been affected by the same factors which influence gastroenteritis mortality, particularly if the diagnostic difficulties at the beginning of life are considered. These two groups of causes of death made only moderate contributions to the mortality decline.

Some of the specific causes of death, such as measles, are even today subject to significant fluctuations from year to year, which makes the interpretation of the percentage changes difficult. However, all of them seem to have contributed, in varying degrees, to the mortality decline. The large changes observed from period to period for malaria and tetanus were consistent with evidence reviewed later. Particularly interesting was the very high contribution that meningitis appears to have made to the mortality decline. (I will say more about these specific diseases when I evaluate the probable causes of mortality decline.)

Using the data in table 15, we can conclude that most of Havana's mortality decline resulted from changes in causes of death of infectious origin. Between 55 and 65 percent of the mortality decline in the City of Havana was produced by reductions in the rates for respiratory tuberculosis; other infectious and parasitic dieseases; influenza, pneumonia, and bronchitis; and diarrhea, gastritis, and enteritis. Actually, the percentage decline from diseases due to microorganisms was even higher, since complications of an infection produced many of the deaths ascribed to cardiovascular diseases, complications of pregnancy, certain degenerative diseases, certain diseases of infancy, accidents and violence, and the "all other and unknown" category. These results are in full agreement with the standard pattern of mortality decline recorded in many countries.

Table 14
Age-Sex-Standardized Cause-Specific Death Rates, Municipality of Havana
(Per 100,000 Population)

Cause of Death	Census Dates					
	1901	1907	1919	1931	1943	1953
Respiratory tuberculosis	360.8	379.0	344.1	164.3	177.0	41.3
Other infectious and parasitic diseases	262.3	222.4	119.9	58.5	74.8	10.6
Malignant and benign tumors	105.7	139.0	186.9	147.8	170.2	176.2
Cardiovascular diseases	675.2	778.7	760.0	536.6	406.3	359.1
Influenza, pneumonia, bronchitis	176.4	178.1	168.8	145.6	113.0	35.4
Diarrhea, gastritis, enteritis	350.8	181.0	227.6	135.0	82.5	23.2
Certain degenerative diseases	126.5	112.8	173.0	143.4	100.7	65.5
Complications of pregnancy	17.7	20.4	23.0	14.4	6.5	1.7
Certain diseases of infancy	36.8	55.7	29.5	18.3	21.0	25.4
Accidents and violence	66.0	81.6	101.7	97.5	60.2	58.9
All other and unknown causes	303.0	301.0	236.0	241.2	222.1	159.8
All causes	2,481.2	2,449.7	2,370.5	1,702.6	1,434.3	957.1
Other infectious and parasitic diseases						
Scarlet fever	1.2	1.1	0.2	—	—	—
Whooping cough	1.4	6.1	0.7	0.6	0.4	—
Measles	1.4	7.6	0.2	1.8	0.4	0.2
Diphtheria	8.4	13.8	2.8	6.3	3.5	0.1
Dysentery	4.4	1.5	0.8	0.6	3.5	0.1
Nonrespiratory tuberculosis	29.1	36.1	21.6	11.4	12.3	2.4
Enteric fever	30.8	30.7	31.6	8.2	23.4	2.4
Malaria	58.2	7.6	5.8	0.9	1.5	—

Table 14—*Continued*

Cause of Death	Census Dates					
	1901	1907	1919	1931	1943	1953
Other infectious and parasitic diseases (continued)						
Syphilis	12.1	11.2	12.2	8.4	11.5	4.4
Meningitis	81.6	75.7	21.2	6.0	11.8	3.7
Tetanus	40.3	12.4	5.8	2.4	5.8	4.6
Certain degenerative diseases						
Nephritis	71.4	69.7	124.2	86.8	53.4	22.8
All other and unknown causes						
Old age	32.4	40.9	25.7	18.8	17.7	10.2
Appendicitis	14.7	14.8	17.5	21.6	11.7	2.0

Source: Cuban censuses and vital statistics.

Note: The rates have been standardized to the age-sex structure of the 1943 population. A dash indicates that no deaths were attributed to the specified cause during that year. Because of problems associated with the classification of certain diseases in 1901 and 1953, the sum of the individual age-sex-standardized cause-specific death rates under the rubric "other infectious and parasitic diseases" exceeds the overall rate for this group as a whole. In 1901 the problem is related to adapting the originally established classification of causes of death to the new classification introduced with the first revision of the International List of Causes of Death. The problem with the 1953 data is related to changes in the classification of meningitis and tetanus. The resultant biases are minor and do not affect the interpretation of secular changes.

Table 15
Contribution of Each Cause-Group or Cause of Death to Mortality Decline, City of Havana
(Percentages)

Cause-Group	Both Sexes		Males		Females	
	1901-1953	1907-1953	1901-1953	1907-1953	1901-1953	1907-1953
Respiratory tuberculosis	21.0	22.6	18.2	21.8	24.5	23.3
Other infectious and parasitic diseases	16.5	14.2	16.8	17.7	16.1	11.0
Malignant and benign tumors	-4.6	-2.5	-5.3	-4.2	-3.8	-0.9
Cardiovascular diseases	20.7	28.1	22.8	27.4	18.1	28.8
Influenza, pneumonia, bronchitis	9.2	9.6	10.2	10.0	8.0	9.1
Diarrhea, gastritis, enteritis	21.5	10.6	20.9	10.8	22.2	10.3
Certain degenerative diseases	4.0	3.2	5.8	3.5	1.7	2.9
Complications of pregnancy	1.0	1.2	—	—	2.4	2.4
Certain diseases of infancy	0.8	2.0	0.8	2.1	0.7	2.0
Accidents and violence	0.5	1.5	0.7	2.3	0.1	0.8
All other and unknown causes	9.4	9.5	9.0	8.5	9.9	10.3
All causes	100.0	100.0	100.0	100.0	100.0	100.0
Other infectious and parasitic diseases						
Scarlet fever	.08	.07	.07	—	.09	.14
Whooping cough	.09	.41	.11	.48	.07	.33
Measles	.08	.49	.11	.52	.03	.47
Diphtheria	.54	.91	.58	1.14	.50	.70
Dysentery	.27	.08	.32	.19	.21	-.02
Nonrespiratory tuberculosis	1.75	2.26	1.09	2.89	2.59	1.67
Enteric fever	1.86	1.89	1.87	2.97	1.86	.89
Malaria	3.82	.51	3.91	.88	3.70	.16
Syphilis	.50	.45	.66	.51	.30	.40

Table 15—*Continued*

Cause-Group	Both Sexes		Males		Females	
	1901-1953	1907-1953	1901-1953	1907-1953	1901-1953	1907-1953
Other infectious and parasitic diseases (continued)						
Meningitis	5.11	4.82	4.85	5.66	5.43	4.05
Tetanus	2.34	.53	2.90	.94	1.63	.14
Certain degenerative diseases						
Nephritis	3.19	3.14	4.27	3.15	1.83	3.14
All other and unknown causes						
Old age	1.46	2.06	1.01	2.26	2.02	2.82
Appendicitis	.83	.86	.79	.87	.89	.85

Source: Table 14.

Note: A dash signifies no deaths reported.

Cause-of-Death Components of the Mortality Decline in Each Age Group

To ascertain the extent to which each cause or group of causes of death contributed to the mortality decline in each age-sex group, I have computed for Havana the declines in mortality for each cause as a percentage of the total decline from all causes within each age-sex group.[8] Table 16 summarizes these percentage contributions.

Infancy (under one year of age)

About 40 percent of the mortality decline in infancy resulted from a reduction in deaths attributed to diarrhea, gastritis, and enteritis. A reduction in the incidence of other diseases of infectious origin produced an additional 40 percent of the decline. Of these infectious diseases, meningitis and tetanus were the greatest contributors.

Ages One to Four

At these ages the diarrhea, gastritis, and enteritis group remained as one of the leading contributors to the mortality decline (approximately 25 percent), but its contribution was exceeded by that of other infectious and parasitic diseases (approximately 40 percent) and almost equaled by that of influenza, pneumonia, and bronchitis (approximately 25 percent). Meningitis, among the infectious diseases, contributed almost the same percentage declines as those attributed to influenza, pneumonia, and bronchitis. Other diseases that appeared to be important contributors to the decline were epidemic maladies, such as measles, that even today are characterized by their cyclical recurrence. Already by these early ages, nonrespiratory tuberculosis was contributing to the mortality decline.

Ages Five to Fourteen

Together, the other infectious and parasitic diseases and respiratory tuberculosis accounted for between 50 and 65 percent of the decline in this age group. Accidents and violence contributed significantly to the decline, particularly for males. Meningitis lost much of its importance, but other infectious diseases, such as enteric fevers (typhoid and paratyphoid) and diphtheria, continued as substantial elements in the decline.

Ages Fifteen to Twenty-Nine

Respiratory tuberculosis reached its highest percentage contribution to the mortality decline in this age group because of the high tuberculosis mortality rates among young adults and the relatively low mortality from other causes at these ages. The other infectious and parasitic diseases continued their pattern of decreasing contribution with advancing age, and declines in mortality from cardiovascular diseases became important in this age group. The enteric fevers alone, among the specific infectious diseases (with the exception of nonrespiratory tuberculosis), continued to contribute significantly to the mortality decline.

Ages Thirty to Forty-Four

Respiratory tuberculosis remained the main contributor to the mortality decline. The other infectious and parasitic diseases (particularly for males) and cardiovascular diseases were also important at these ages. Cardiovascular diseases rapidly increased their share with advancing age. Certain degenerative diseases began to acquire importance, with nephritis alone accounting for approximately 5 percent of the decline.

Ages Forty-Five to Fifty-Nine

In this age group, declines in cardiovascular diseases almost equaled those resulting from tuberculosis. The contribution of other infectious and parasitic diseases continued to diminish, and the incidence of malignant and benign tumors increased. Certain degenerative diseases remained important contributors to the decline, with nephritis still a significant factor.

Ages above Sixty

Above age sixty, the importance of respiratory tuberculosis and of the other infectious and parasitic diseases as factors in the decline of mortality became relatively minor, except in the case of males with respiratory tuberculosis. Cardiovascular diseases accounted for most of the decline at these ages, and mortality attributed to tumors increased. Nor surprisingly, deaths under the rubric of old age declined substantially in these population groups. Fairly large declines attributed to influenza, pneumonia, and bronchitis, in particular for males, were recorded above age sixty. Some increases were observable for certain degenerative diseases. Unquestionably, diagnostic difficulties at these ages tended to produce some irregular patterns in the mortality decline by cause.

Table 16

Mortality Declines for Each Cause-Group as Percentage of Total Decline from All Causes, Municipality of Havana, 1907-1953

Cause-Group	Under 1		1-4		5-14		15-29		30-44		45-59		60-74		75 and over	
	M	F	M	F	M	F	M	F	M	F	M	F	M	F	M	F
Respiratory tuberculosis	-0.1	—	0.2	0.7	25.6	25.2	46.0	60.4	34.1	36.7	40.2	29.8	24.3	8.2	6.1	-0.7
Other infectious and parasitic diseases	28.0	21.8	37.6	42.0	49.3	26.7	22.5	9.7	14.1	5.0	10.3	4.5	4.8	3.5	4.4	1.7
Malignant and benign tumors	-0.1	—	-0.4	-1.2	-6.1	-2.9	-3.4	1.5	2.0	-6.7	-9.8	-6.7	-37.0	-12.5	-13.8	-7.5
Cardiovascular diseases	0.4	0.3	-0.2	0.3	-0.3	2.9	6.5	6.9	19.0	18.4	34.4	38.9	88.6	76.6	76.6	75.1
Influenza, pneumonia, bronchitis	12.8	11.9	31.6	21.8	4.3	15.0	4.6	5.4	5.6	6.8	4.8	11.8	16.4	10.8	14.0	3.3
Diarrhea, gastritis, enteritis	38.9	42.3	24.9	23.9	4.8	5.8	1.8	2.4	1.9	2.9	4.3	3.7	6.4	6.6	3.1	4.4
Certain degenerative diseases	0.6	—	-0.1	1.2	0.0	5.6	4.1	2.3	8.2	7.8	6.6	5.2	-0.1	1.3	-1.4	-3.0
Complications of pregnancy	—						—	8.2	—	4.7	—	0.4				
Certain diseases of infancy	12.5	15.0														
Accidents and violence	0.3	0.1	1.3	2.7	10.3	1.2	7.0	-0.3	2.5	0.7	4.1	0.5	-3.8	1.6	-1.8	-0.7
All other & unknown causes	6.6	8.6	5.1	8.5	12.1	20.6	10.9	3.5	12.6	10.2	5.0	11.9	0.6	6.5	12.7	27.4
All causes	100.0	100.0	100.0	100.0	100.0	100.0	100.0	100.0	100.0	100.0	100.0	100.0	100.0	100.0	100.0	100.0
Other infectious and parasitic diseases																
Scarlet fever	—	—	—	0.7	—	2.2										
Whooping cough	1.7	1.4	1.8	1.5	0.2	1.1										

Table 16—Continued

Cause-Group	Under 1 M	Under 1 F	1-4 M	1-4 F	5-14 M	5-14 F	15-29 M	15-29 F	30-44 M	30-44 F	45-59 M	45-59 F	60-74 M	60-74 F	75 and over M	75 and over F
Other infectious and parasitic diseases																
Measles	0.3	-0.1	2.8	5.8	1.2	1.1	1.3	—	—	—	—	—	—	—	—	—
Diphtheria	0.5	—	8.9	6.2	7.3	6.2	—	—	—	—	—	—	—	—	—	—
Dysentery	—	—	—	—	—	—	—	—	0.2	-0.1	0.4	—	—	—	1.3	—
Nonrespiratory tuberculosis	1.1	1.4	2.2	3.3	6.3	0.6	4.8	2.3	5.7	2.3	3.2	1.5	1.8	1.2	—	—
Enteric fever	—	—	0.7	0.0	18.8	5.8	10.1	2.4	2.5	0.6	2.8	1.0	—	—	—	—
Malaria	0.7	0.2	0.7	0.7	2.4	1.1	0.2	0.2	1.2	—	0.5	—	0.9	—	2.6	—
Syphilis	0.4	0.8	—	0.4	—	—	0.5	0.2	1.7	0.5	0.4	0.3	-0.3	-0.2	-0.8	1.0
Meningitis	22.3	18.0	19.6	20.8	8.0	2.4	0.1	—	-0.3	-0.1	-0.2	—	—	—	—	—
Tetanus	2.7	1.4	0.2	0.0	3.6	-0.3	0.8	0.3	0.5	-0.1	0.8	-0.1	0.6	-0.2	-0.2	—
Certain degenerative diseases																
Nephritis	0.4	—	0.5	1.4	0.5	4.5	2.3	1.3	4.6	6.5	6.9	6.5	7.6	3.1	0.6	1.0
All other & unknown causes																
Old age	—	—	—	—	—	—	—	—	—	—	—	—	0.6	2.0	15.1	26.4
Appendicitis	—	—	-0.4	0.5	1.5	-0.5	2.6	1.2	1.6	2.2	1.2	1.6	0.6	—	-0.4	—

Source: Cuban censuses and vital statistics.

Note: A dash signifies that no deaths were attributed to that cause during that year; zero signifies that less than one-tenth of one percent of the change resulted from that cause.

International Comparisons of Components of Secular Changes in Mortality by Age Groups and Causes of Death

The pattern of mortality decline by cause and age conforms closely to that observed in other populations, with the younger age groups experiencing substantially greater declines in mortality from infectious causes. The age structure (Havana's) used to examine these changes explains some of the observed deviations. As in other urban populations, Havana's population was heavily concentrated in ages fifteen to sixty-four, with only a small proportion of the total under age five. The less-dependable data for the whole country (analyzed in the next chapter) suggest, however, that the mortality changes experienced by Cuba followed the trends recorded elsewhere. In Cuba as a whole, as in Havana, the causes of death that appear to have declined the most were respiratory tuberculosis; other infectious and parasitic diseases; cardiovascular diseases; influenza, pneumonia, and bronchitis; and diarrhea, gastritis, and enteritis. These are the same cause-groups identified by Preston as the major contributors to mortality declines in his study of 165 populations representing forty-three nations at different points in time.[9] The changes I have described here for Cuba also follow closely those reported for Chile by Hugo Behm, in what is perhaps the only other major study available of long-term trends of mortality by cause for another Latin American country.[10] Although the cause-groups used in the Chilean analysis do not exactly match those used in this study, and the time periods are not the same, both sets show basically similar patterns of change in cause-specific mortality. More importantly, marked downturns for certain causes, particularly at about the time of the Second World War, appear to have occurred simultaneously in both countries, which suggests that similar determining causes may have been involved. How the timing of these changes relates to causative factors behind the trend of mortality decline in Havana and in Cuba is the subject of the next chapter.

6. The Decline of Mortality from Specific Causes

This chapter examines the factors that contributed to the decline of mortality rates for each of the groups of causes considered in the preceding chapter, against the background of political, economic, social, and medical developments sketched in Chapter 4. The discussion refers primarily to the experience of the City of Havana during the first half of this century, but will also take into account the experience of non-Havana Cuba, within the limits of the available data.

Tuberculosis

As we have seen, tuberculosis (respiratory and nonrespiratory combined) contributed approximately 25 percent to the mortality decline in the City of Havana from 1901 (or 1907) to 1953. Furthermore, the largest percentage contributions occurred at ages fifteen to fifty-nine, ages in which the greatest percentage of the population of the city was concentrated and in which tuberculosis mortality rates were higher than in other age groups.

The causes of the very significant declines in tuberculosis mortality throughout the world since the nineteenth century have been amply discussed in the literature.[1] Researchers generally believe that most of the decline until the middle of the present century resulted from improvements in social and economic conditions, especially in the areas of nutrition, housing, and working conditions, and from the reduction of contagion resulting from the isolation of infected persons in sanatoriums, starting in the late nineteenth century. Other more-or-less effective methods used for the prevention and treatment of tuberculosis during the period under discussion included the pasteurization of milk and the elimination of tuberculous cattle as means of combating the bovine forms of the disease (since the 1880s); lung-collapse therapy, used with more questionable effectiveness against the respiratory forms (also since the 1880s); and the traditional therapy of bed rest and a high-protein diet (practiced since the second half of the nineteenth century). The BCG vaccine, available since 1921, was apparently not used to any great extent in many countries until two or three decades later. Since 1947 very effective methods of chemotherapy and immunization against tuberculosis have been developed.

Three key questions must be raised when attempting to assess the impact of any specific measure on the trend of mortality from tuberculosis or any other disease: (1) When did specific measures become available, wherever they originated? (2) How effective were these measures? and (3) When and to what extent were available measures put into effect in the area under study? The third question is especially important for developing countries, where few of the sanitary and therapeutic advances originated.

As noted in Chapter 3, the United States military government tried at the beginning of the present century to combat tuberculosis in Cuba by establishing a commission to investigate possible measures for reducing the propagation of the disease in cattle. In 1907 public funds were allocated for the construction of Cuba's first hospital for tuberculous patients (in Havana), and for the establishment of tuberculosis clinics in the capital. In 1910 additional funds were approved for the expansion of the tuberculosis sanatorium (to 150 beds).[2] There is considerable discussion in the literature of this period regarding the measures for assuring a purer supply of milk, such as pasteurization, the proper handling of milk on dairy farms, and sanitary procedures for its distribution.[3]

There is some evidence that as early as 1928, the BCG vaccine was used in Cuba, but it was given only to the newborn of tuberculous mothers.[4] In 1927 the National Bureau of Statistics and Information was created, having as one of its major functions the communication of known measures of tuberculosis control.[5]

In 1936, apparently in the belief that earlier efforts had been inadequate, the National Council of Tuberculosis was instituted. It was to educate the public in ways of avoiding contagion, to furnish aid for people who had contracted the disease and to develop facilities for isolating them, and to protect infants who had been exposed to infection. In the following year, tuberculosis clinics were established in all provincial capitals that did not already have them, and a nationwide tuberculosis survey was carried out, especially in hospitals, asylums, public schools and nurseries, and in slum areas. The survey employed X-ray examinations, tuberculin tests, and other laboratory examinations.[6]

The 1943 census summary reported that in that year there were four major hospitals either fully or partially dedicated to tuberculosis treatment, as well as local dispensaries in many municipalities, and that a large facility for treatment of tuberculosis was under construction in Las Villas Province.[7] World-wide evidence and fairly reliable statistical data for the City of Havana indicate a pronounced drop in the tuberculosis mortality rate between 1943 and 1953 and strongly suggest that modern chemotherapy for this disease was introduced into the country at the end of the Second World War.

Table 14 shows that the rates of tuberculosis mortality in Havana did not change very significantly between 1901 and 1919.[8] However, between 1919 and 1931 the rates for both respiratory and nonrespiratory tuberculosis were reduced by approximately 50 percent. From 1931 to 1943 the rates changed little, but between 1943 and 1953 the rates for both types of tuberculosis declined by approximately 75 percent. Table 17 demonstrates the extent to which cause-specific mortality had declined by 1931 and by 1943. The percentage declines are expressed as a percent of the total decline within each cause from 1901 to 1953. As table 17 shows, close to 60 percent of the decline in tuberculosis mortality between 1901 and 1953 had occurred by 1931.

The Cuban evidence suggests that any direct impact of medical advances, allowing for a substantial lag in effects of preventive and curative measures, can have been only minimal by 1931. We can almost discount the effects of the BCG vaccine, since it was probably not used to any great extent until years later. The isolation and treatment of tuberculosis patients may have had some effect after 1910 in Havana, but it is highly unlikely that isolation and treatment had any substantial influence outside of Havana before the late 1920s, when tuberculosis services were first extended to other parts of the country.

Since underregistration of deaths was prevalent outside Havana, especially in the rural areas and for infants, it is impossible to determine statistically to what extent the observed pattern of tuberculosis mortality decline for Havana was duplicated in the rest of the country. However, we can get some indication by studying the patterns of change in the percentage distribution of deaths by cause.[9]

Figure 8 shows the percentages of all registered deaths attributed to respiratory tuberculosis in the municipality of Havana, in all of Cuba, and in non-Havana Cuba in the years for which data are available between 1902 and 1953. Two features stand out: the relatively high percentages of deaths attributed to respiratory tuberculosis in the municipality of Havana,[10] and the similar shapes of the three curves. The similarity of the curves shows a gradual decline in the relative importance of tuberculosis as a cause of death in all three areas, until after the end of the Second World War, when the decline accelerated markedly.[11]

The evidence presented above strongly suggests that economic factors

Table 17
Declines in Age-Sex-Standardized Cause-Specific Death Rates,
Municipality of Havana
(Percentages)

Cause-Group	1931[a]	1943[a]
Respiratory tuberculosis	61.5	57.5
Other infectious and parasitic diseases	81.0	74.5
Malignant and benign tumors	*	*
Cardiovascular diseases	43.8	85.0
Influenza, pneumonia, bronchitis	21.8	45.0
Diarrhea, gastritis, enteritis	65.9	81.9
Certain degenerative diseases	*	42.4
Complications of pregnancy	21.1	70.2
Certain diseases of infancy	*	*
Accidents and violence	*	82.0
All other and unknown causes	43.2	56.6
All causes	51.1	68.7
Other infectious and parasitic diseases		
Scarlet fever	100.0	100.0
Whooping cough	53.7	67.6
Measles	*	83.5
Diphtheria	25.5	58.9
Dysentery	90.5	19.9
Nonrespiratory tuberculosis	66.3	63.1
Enteric fever	79.7	26.4
Malaria	98.4	97.5
Syphilis	47.8	7.0
Meningitis	97.1	89.6
Tetanus	100.0[b]	96.6
Certain degenerative diseases		
Nephritis	*	79.3
All other and unknown causes		
Old age	61.3	65.9
Appendicitis	*	23.6

Source: This study.

[a] Calculated as a percentage of the total decline within each cause from 1901 to 1953.

[b] In later years the cause-specific rate was higher than in this year.

* The rates were actually higher in this year than at the beginning of the period.

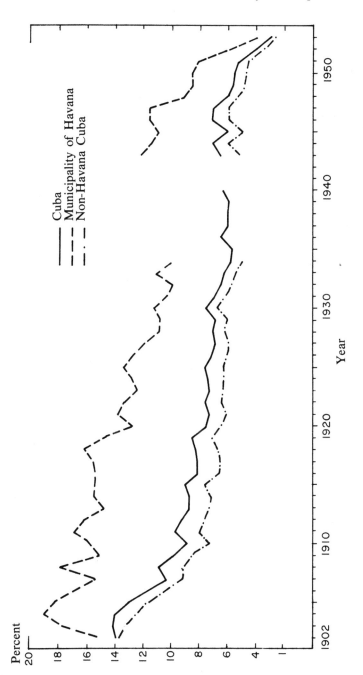

Figure 8. Deaths Attributed to Respiratory Tuberculosis

Source: Cuban vital statistics; tables 54 and 55, this study.

played an important role in the decline of mortality from tuberculosis. The trends of tuberculosis mortality seem to parallel the trend of per capita rice consumption, which serves as a proxy for changes in levels of nutrition (see Chapter 4). Since rice imports were heavily dependent on the availability of foreign exchange, the amount of rice imported was largely determined by the levels of national income. In view of the fact that Cuba is an island country, largely dependent on imported food, these observations tend to confirm the postulated relationship between tuberculosis mortality and nutrition.

Favorable economic conditions in the years before 1931 may have contributed to the decline of tuberculosis mortality by facilitating the development of government- and privately funded medical facilities. The very interesting possibility emerges that the further expansion of government-funded medical facilities during the mid- to late 1930s and the early 1940s was not sufficient to induce further declines in tuberculosis mortality, in the absence of favorable economic conditions (and with a likely deterioration in nutrition). However, it seems almost certain that the isolation of the sick and the dissemination of information concerning tuberculosis were also important prior to the 1930s. Advances that would be expected under favorable economic conditions in areas such as housing and popular education probably were also influential. After the Second World War, in contrast, the tuberculosis mortality trend appears to have been largely dissociated from socioeconomic factors.

The evidence, then, suggests that the tuberculosis mortality decline in Cuba up to the time of the Great Depression was produced primarily by improvements in nutrition, which were directly dependent on economic conditions, because much of the food consumed in the country was imported. I attribute secondary importance to other variables that appear to have contributed to the decline of this disease. This conclusion is similar to that of McKeown and associates with reference to England and Wales.[12] What is peculiar to Cuba is that the mortality decline from tuberculosis appears to have been more responsive to economic conditions, since, in Cuba, unlike in England and Wales, a continuous secular trend of economic growth did not hold. Hence, in Cuba, when the economy was growing, tuberculosis mortality was declining, but when the economy stagnated, so did mortality decline from that disease. After 1947 the resumed acceleration of tuberculosis mortality decline seems to have been independent of economic factors, although it is true that economic conditions were improving by that time.

Other Infectious and Parasitic Diseases

This group includes smallpox, yellow fever, scarlet fever, whooping cough, measles, diphtheria, dysentery, nonrespiratory tuberculosis, typhoid and paratyphoid fevers, malaria, syphilis, meningitis, and tetanus. An important share of the mortality decline in Cuba, as in other countries during modern times, has been due to the diminished prevalence and lethality of diseases in this group.

At the beginning of this century, mortality from the group of infectious and parasitic diseases was high in Havana and higher yet elsewhere in Cuba, where sanitary conditions were poorer. Figure 9 depicts the trends between 1902 and 1953 in yearly percentages of all deaths attributed to diseases in this group in Cuba as a whole, in Havana, and in the rest of the country. Throughout the period, the "other infectious and parasitic" diseases accounted for a larger proportionate share of deaths outside Havana than within. This understates the relative disadvantage of the population outside Havana in mortality from these diseases, since a larger proportion of the non-Havana than of the Havana population consisted of infants and young children—age groups in which the incidence of most infectious and parasitic diseases is greatest—and since there was greater underregistration of infant deaths outside Havana.

The nearly parallel trends of all three curves in figure 9 imply that the rest of the country followed Havana closely in the pace and timing of decrease in mortality from this group of diseases. There were two periods of especially rapid decline: one between 1902 and approximately 1910 and another after 1945. We can attribute the steep decline of the curves during the earlier period to the sanitary reforms instituted at that time, including the mosquito control campaign. A primary factor during the later period was certainly the introduction of chemotherapy. Explosive recurrences of epidemic malaria explain the significant reversals of the trend, marked by the peaks in 1921 and in 1934.

Malaria

Although Cuba is located within the world-wide band of malaria endemicity, reliable data indicate that malaria has always been less important as a cause of death in Cuba than in many other tropical countries. A country-wide malaria survey carried out between 1938 and 1941 by the public health authorities of Cuba, in cooperation with a medical team of the Rockefeller Foundation, supports this interpretation.[13] The team examined 90,767 children, from urban and rural areas in all the regions in the country, for evidence of clinical splenomegaly. Half of the sample had their blood examined to study the prevalence of malaria parasites. The results provided two widely used indices of malaria prevalence, the spleen and the parasite rates, which can be contrasted with similar data from other countries in

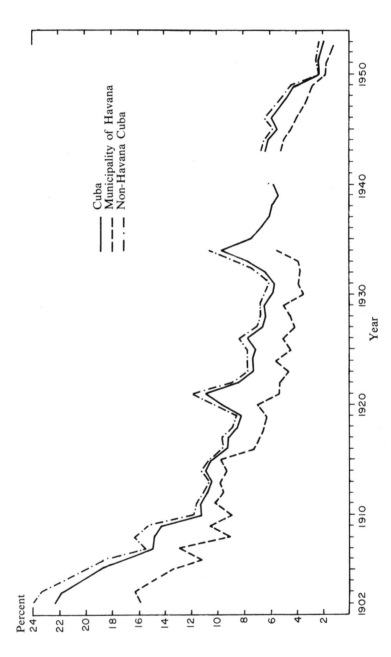

Figure 9. Deaths Attributed to Other Infectious and Parasitic Diseases

order to assess the relative importance of malaria in Cuba.[14]

The authors of the Cuban malaria survey report concluded that the disease was not endemic in a major portion of the country and that it was only moderately endemic in a limited number of areas. Compared with other tropical countries, the importance of malaria in Cuba was minor. Since malaria was not endemic in much of the country, large epidemics occasionally occurred, and localized epidemic outbursts happened practically every year. The report attributed Cuba's relatively low malarial endemicity primarily to the nature of its soil (Matanzas clay), which allows rapid drainage of rain water. Many of the localized epidemics resulted from man-made conditions that were easily correctable.[15]

The traditional prophylaxis against malaria has been quinine, known for centuries. Since the connection between mosquitoes and malaria was made, mosquito control by swamp drainage, spreading of larvicides over stagnant waters, and protection of water deposits has been widely used. Screening homes is also an effective control. Since the Second World War, residual insecticides, such as DDT, have been used extensively. Increasingly since the start of the chemotherapeutic era, chemical compounds have been used against the disease, although in many cases the response has been poor.[16] No effective immunization measures have been developed yet.

Table 18 shows the declining trend in annual numbers of registered deaths attributed to malaria in Havana and in Cuba as a whole, from 1902 to 1953. In Havana, the contribution of the decline of malaria to the total decline of mortality during this period is estimated at about 4 percent. However, most of the decline occurred before 1907. The antimosquito campaign, initiated during the early 1900s as part of the effort to eradicate yellow fever, surely affected the incidence of malaria. The return of peacetime conditions may also have played a part, since it appears that malaria attained epidemic proportions during the war years and immediately after.

The increase in malaria deaths around 1920 was associated with the arrival of tens of thousands of laborers from Jamaica and Haiti. These laborers, who brought malaria parasites with them, went to work in malaria-endemic areas and spread the parasites to the rest of the population.[17] Because there was a labor shortage, the immigration laws were relaxed, which permitted the entrance of less-healthy aliens from areas where sanitary conditions were poor (for example, Haiti) and of low-health population strata from other countries, such as Jamaica.[18]

Furthermore, the enforcement of the port-quarantine laws was neglected. Table 18 shows that around 1920 the incidence of measles and smallpox, as well as of malaria, increased dramatically, but after the laws requiring inspection of arriving aliens and mandatory vaccination against smallpox were tightened, not another death from smallpox was recorded. The relative decline in malaria mortality was produced by reinstitution of the antimosquito campaign and the wide distribution of free quinine.[19]

The second peak in malaria mortality, recorded in 1934, was associated with excessive rains in that year. Deterioration of economic conditions may also have contributed to the outbreak, since the distribution of free quinine and drainage efforts may have been curtailed. After 1935 the antimosquito campaign was again intensified and led to a substantial reduction in the number of registered malaria deaths. After 1945 the decline in malaria mortality suggests that residual insecticides were used. It is important to realize that DDT contributed to the reduction of malaria mortality only after it had already declined significantly.

Measles and Whooping Cough

The trends of mortality from measles and whooping cough in Cuba, as in other countries, show the patterns of moderate endemicity with occasional epidemic outbursts that are characteristic of these two diseases. Table 18 shows the recorded annual number of deaths from measles in Havana and in the whole of Cuba from 1902 to 1953. Estimates are that the diminishing incidence of measles and of whooping cough each contributed less than 1 percent to the total decline of mortality in Havana during the period.

In the case of England and Wales, McKeown, Record, and Turner attributed most of the decline of whooping cough mortality to "reduced exposure as a result of improved hygiene and related measures," the case with most of the airborne diseases.[20] Abram Benenson supports this conclusion and also claims that active immunization, as opposed to passive, has been proved effective against the disease.[21] In any event, immunization has only been possible since the early 1950s.

With regard to measles, McKeown, Record, and Turner stated that

effective specific measures against measles have only recently become available in the form of immunization and they can have had no significant effect on the trend of the death rate [in England and Wales]. However, mortality from the disease was attributable largely to invasion by secondary organisms, which have been treated by chemotherapy since 1935. Epidemiological evidence suggests that nutrition plays an important part in the individual's reaction to measles. [In England and Wales] . . . infection rates were high and approximately the same in all social classes; but mortality rates were much greater among the poor than among the well to do. Similarly, in developing countries today, there is little doubt that the devastating effects of measles are associated with low living standards. The explanation accepted by most epidemiologists with extensive experience of measles is that although infection rates are largely independent of social circumstances, the mortality that results from the infection is determined mainly by nutritional state.[22]

Evidence for the United States supports this interpretation and indicates the strong association that measles has with other diseases and with nutrition.[23]

Since measles and whooping cough have been found to respond only to the drugs available since the 1930s, their earlier declines in Cuba must have resulted from other factors, such as general improvement in sanitary conditions and better popular understanding of the causes and consequences of infectious and communicable diseases.[24] The data in table 18 infer that the introduction of sulfonamides in the late 1930s played a significant role in the decline of measles mortality, more clearly marked in Havana than in the rest of the country. There is some evidence of attempts made in Havana in the late 1930s and early 1940s to control whooping cough morbidity and mortality by means of a locally developed antitoxin, but evidently it was of no value.[25]

Dysentery and Enteric Fevers

Dysentery and typhoid and paratyphoid fevers result mainly from the use of contaminated water, although these infections can also be transmitted by the ingestion of contaminated seafood and vegetables, unpasteurized milk, and by personal contact.[26] Bacillary dysentery is a relatively mild disease in temperate climates, but it is an important cause of death in less-developed tropical and subtropical countries, where malnutrition is common.[27] The decline of mortality from the enteric fevers in European countries has been attributed primarily to the extension of hygienic measures begun in the nineteenth century, such as the purification of water, sanitary disposal of sewage, and improved food handling. Effective treatment of these diseases (by chloramphenicol) was not available until 1950.[28] Certain antimicrobial drugs are effective in the treatment of dysentery, but no effective method of immunization against either dysentery or the enteric fevers has yet been found.[29]

In Havana, the decline of enteric fever mortality contributed between 2 and 3 percent to the total mortality decline during the first half of this century, while the decline of dysentery contributed less than 1 percent. Since no effective specific measures against the enteric fevers became available until 1950, and none, even today, has proved very effective against dysentery, most of the mortality decline from these two disease groups

Table 18
Deaths Attributed to Malaria, Measles, and Smallpox
(Absolute Numbers)

Year	Malaria		Measles		Smallpox	
	Havana	Cuba	Havana	Cuba	Havana	Cuba
1902	77	1,546	4	6	—	3
1903	51	1,204	9	12	—	—
1904	44	1,079	25	33	1	1
1905	32	1,100	73	184	—	4
1906	26	1,147	16	163	—	—
1907	23	925	33	117	—	—
1908	19	730	13	62	—	—
1909	6	745	51	113	—	—
1910	15	617	6	83	—	—
1911	12	526	21	99	—	—
1912	4	492	3	24	—	—
1913	5	447	33	70	—	—
1914	4	454	13	121	1	1
1915	4	542	1	22	—	3
1916	14	715	33	189	—	—
1917	5	648	11	148	—	—
1918	8	480	3	20	—	—
1919	19	436	1	3	2	3
1920	20	956	46	362	1	11
1921	23	1,608	4	130	—	316
1922	35	864	1	5	1	158
1923	29	656	—	1	—	2
1924	16	636	2	17	—	2
1925	19	794	31	153	—	—
1926	17	961	12	187	—	—
1927	12	686	7	44	—	—
1928	17	462	5	16	—	—
1929	6	334	32	72	—	—
1930	5	320	—	17	—	—
1931	5	412	11	22	—	—
1932	16	704	1	53	—	—

Table 18—*Continued*

Year	Malaria		Measles		Smallpox	
	Havana	Cuba	Havana	Cuba	Havana	Cuba
1933	19	1,305	3	50	—	—
1934	55	1,929	—	30	—	—
1935	n.a.	1,068	n.a.	150	—	—
1936	n.a.	686	n.a.	18	—	—
1937	n.a.	450	n.a.	16	—	—
1938	n.a.	276	n.a.	42	—	—
1939	n.a.	180	n.a.	32	—	—
1940	9	194	6	42	—	—
1941	n.a.	n.a.	n.a.	n.a.	n.a.	n.a.
1942	n.a.	n.a.	n.a.	n.a.	n.a.	n.a.
1943	10	328	3	18	—	—
1944	10	351	4	74	—	—
1945	5	342	1	33	—	—
1946	2	266	—	22	—	—
1947	7	201	3	76	—	—
1948	2	180	5	39	—	—
1949	—	155	3	25	—	—
1950	1	92	—	35	—	—
1951	—	61	8	52	—	—
1952	4	66	4	42	—	—
1953	—	44	2	18	—	—

Source: Cuban vital statistics.

Notes: A dash signifies no deaths attributed to this cause during the year. N.A. signifies no data available.

probably resulted from improvement in the water supply.

Meningitis

Mortality from meningitis, of all the diseases in the "other infectious and parasitic" group, appears to have declined most in Havana. About 5 percent of the total mortality decline in the city between 1902 and 1953 is attributed to the decline of this disease. However, this estimate is uncertain because of the difficulty of diagnosing meningitis, especially in infants and young children, among whom the disease is common. The incidence of meningitis mortality in Havana is probably exaggerated in the statistics, because deaths due to other causes are often assigned to this disease.

The American Public Health Association feels that the inculcation of good habits of personal hygiene and the prevention of overcrowding are among the most effective measures against the spread of meningitis.[30] Some of the antibiotics, penicillin in particular, are known to alleviate its most serious consequences. It is remarkable that in Havana, 70 to 74 percent of the recorded decrease in meningitis mortality had occurred by 1919, before any effective method of treatment was available. This decline corresponds with the period in which yellow fever was almost completely eradicated and with the two decades in which nonrespiratory tuberculosis first started to decline significantly in the city. These observations suggest that the label "meningitis" may have been used as a convenient category in which to place many infant deaths for which the causes of death were uncertain. Most of the decline in mortality attributed to meningitis probably resulted from improvements in environmental sanitation.

Tetanus

Tetanus is a common cause of death in rural areas of developing countries, especially tetanus neonatorum, which frequently results from the application of unsterilized dressings to the umbilical cord.[31] A toxoid against tetanus was developed in 1924, but was not extensively used, at least in the United States, until 1933.[32] Some of the most effective measures contributing to the decline of mortality from tetanus have been the licensing of midwives and the educating of mothers, relatives, and attendants in the practice of asepsis in treating the umbilical cord.[33]

Tetanus contributed over 2 percent to the total mortality decline in Havana from 1901 to 1953. As in the case of malaria, most of the decline in tetanus mortality took place between 1901 and 1907, and can be directly traced to a decline in the prevalence of tetanus neonatorum.[34] During the years of the first American intervention (1898-1902), as well as during the first few years of the republic, the sanitation authorities distributed free septic packages for the healing of the umbilical cord and widely publicized and described how this easily avoidable cause of death could be eliminated.[35]

Scarlet Fever and Diphtheria

McKeown and associates have concluded that most of the decline in mortality from scarlet fever in England and Wales was due to weakening of the virulence of the infective organism. Effective specific treatment for this disease has been available only since prontosil was introduced in 1935.[36]

With regard to diphtheria, a consensus is found in the literature on the effectiveness of the antitoxin that has been available since 1890, and on the effectiveness of immunization, available since 1941. As in the case of scarlet fever, it is possible that changes in the virulence of the diphtheria agents may have been involved in the mortality decline.[37]

In Havana, diphtheria and scarlet fever each contributed about 1 percent to the decline of mortality during the first half of this century. By 1931, some years before prontosil became available, mortality from scarlet fever had been eliminated (see tables 14 and 17), although the prevalence of the disease remained high (almost everyone gets it, usually during childhood). It seems, therefore, that the decline of mortality from scarlet fever in Havana, as in England, Wales, and elsewhere, resulted from weakening of the virulence of the microorganism. The decline of diphtheria mortality was probably due primarily to the gradual distribution of the antitoxin, known since 1890. The diphtheria antitoxin was distributed gratis by the national sanitation authorities on request.[38]

Syphilis

Preparations of mercury and bismuth have been utilized against syphilis since the nineteenth century; salvarsan, an effective therapeutic agent, became available in 1916; in 1945, penicillin largely replaced the arsenic compounds.[39] Syphilis is estimated to have contributed close to 1 percent to the mortality decline in Havana. However, since many biases affect the recording of syphilis-related deaths, it is difficult to assess properly the secular trend of syphilis mortality.[40] In Havana the disease did not seem to decline substantially until after the appearance of penicillin in 1945, despite the earlier availability of salvarsan and other compounds.

Intestinal Parasites

Although intestinal parasites directly cause few deaths, their debilitating effect contributes significantly to mortality from other causes. A survey of the rural population of Cuba during the late 1940s concerning the prevalence of intestinal parasites provided a clear indication of the poor sanitary conditions in rural parts of the country. This survey found that 86.5 percent of the rural population had intestinal parasites, and that the percentage was even higher among infants.[41] This high incidence of parasites is not surprising if we recall that over 65 percent of all rural dwellings in Cuba still had dirt floors in 1953.

A national campaign against intestinal parasites was initiated in 1946, and laboratories and dispensaries were established in each of the Cuban municipalities.[42] The success of these efforts was facilitated by the development of chemical treatment methods.[43]

In summary, the "other infectious and parasitic" diseases contributed 15 percent to the mortality decline in the City of Havana from 1901 to 1953. About 80 percent of the decline from these diseases combined had occurred by 1931, although hardly any specific measures became available to deal with most of them before that time (the exceptions being smallpox, diphtheria, malaria, and syphilis). Most of the declines in mortality from these diseases in Cuba resulted from the application of sanitary measures developed in other countries. What is peculiar in the Cuban case is that these measures were adopted much earlier than in many other regions of the developing world. The proximity and political and economic ties of Cuba to the United States were important factors in the early implementation of sanitary measures. Another important factor was the relatively high per capita income level attained in Cuba early in the century.

Government decisions and expenditures to improve environmental sanitation, to distribute free live-saving materials (diphtheria antitoxin, smallpox vaccinations, septic packages to reduce neonatorum tetanus mortality), and to disseminate sanitation know-how were paramount in promoting the decline of mortality from these diseases in Havana. Also important were similar private decisions and expenditures, such as membership in the mutualist associations. Undoubtedly, general economic conditions were closely intertwined with these developments. It appears that when economic conditions deteriorated, so did the general-health levels, perhaps because both government and private health expenditures had to be curtailed (for example, the construction of only two aqueducts in the country during the 1930s and the serious outbreak of malaria toward the middle of the decade).

The evidence suggests that what occurred in the city was also taking place in the rest of Cuba, although to a lesser extent and with a substantial lag. The failure to extend the sanitary measures instituted in Havana to the same degree in the rest of the country was the major cause of the differentials in mortality.

Malignant and Benign Tumors

This group shows a constant trend of increase throughout the period in Havana. Improvements in the diagnoses of causes of death and the aging of the city's population produced by declining fertility and substantial migration of adults to the city accounted for this trend. In an older population there is a higher incidence of mortality from malignant and benign tumors. The secular decline in the age-sex-standardized rates of deaths attributed to old age (table 14) suggests that improvement in the diagnosis of causes of death also contributed to the increase in recorded mortality from tumors.

The data in figure 10 show that the increasing secular trend in the percentage of registered deaths ascribed to malignant and benign tumors in Havana was similar to the trend in the rest of the country. The higher percentages of deaths from these causes in the City of Havana were consistent with the greater proportion of the city's population in the older age groups, with a more substantial reduction of deaths from other causes in Havana, and with the concentration of the country's main hospital facilities in the capital. The pronounced upward slope of all three curves after 1945 results from the drastic decline in mortality from infectious diseases after that time, so that the relative share of the degenerative diseases became greater.

Cardiovascular Diseases

Cardiovascular diseases accounted for approximately 20 percent of the decline of mortality in Havana from 1901 to 1953. Even though the age structure of the population in the urban conglomerate magnifies the impact of the mortality decline from cardiovascular diseases, such a large contribution from these diseases appears suspicious. However, a number of factors may explain it.

First, as Samuel Preston, Nathan Keyfitz, and Robert Schoen have indicated, many of the causes of death included under this label are infectious in nature (such as acute endocarditis, rheumatic fever, and rheumatic heart disease).[44] Second, "even when heart disease is not of infectious origin, infectious diseases, particularly those with respiratory complications, can precipitate a cardio-vascular incident."[45] Third, with increasing medical knowledge many deaths which formerly were ascribed to

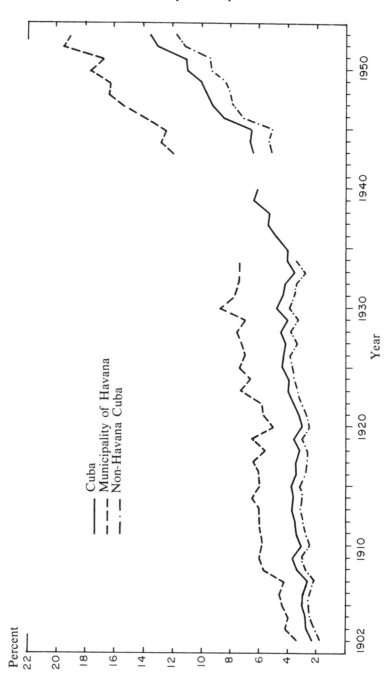

Figure 10. Deaths Attributed to Malignant and Benign Tumors

cardiovascular disease shifted to other categories of cause of death. Finally, there appears to be a strong association between the incidence of many cardiovascular diseases and living conditions—in particular, nutrition.[46]

The data for Havana indicate that mortality from the cardiovascular diseases did not decline until the 1919-1931 period, which suggests that the improvement in economic conditions during the preceding decades influenced somewhat the decline of mortality from these diseases. Between 1931 and 1943, contrary to what was observed with respiratory tuberculosis and the other infectious and parasitic diseases, mortality from cardiovascular diseases continued to decline, as a result of the appearance of the sulfonamides. These drugs are very effective against some of the infectious cardiovascular diseases and against the frequently associated respiratory complications (influenza, pneumonia, and bronchitis). A deceleration in the rate of mortality decline from these causes between 1943 and 1953 suggests that after the appearance of the sulfonamides, only minor advances (probably associated with the use of antibiotics after 1945) were made against cardiovascular mortality. After 1945, the conditions that caused this disease were degenerative, and medical treatment of degenerative ailments had only recently become effective. In 1953 deaths from cardiovascular diseases accounted for over a third of the total death rate, as opposed to about a quarter in 1901, when the overall level of mortality was approximately three times higher.

The increase in the share of mortality attributed to cardiovascular diseases resulted from the relatively greater reduction in mortality from other causes, as well as from the aging of the population due to a decline in fertility. In Havana the percentage increase in cardiovascular diseases was also influenced by a history of migration to the city, and as figure 11 shows, the trend of gradual increase in percentages of all recorded deaths ascribed to cardiovascular diseases has been marked in non-Havana Cuba, as well as in Havana. It is interesting to note the relative narrowing of the gap between the percentages for Havana and non-Havana Cuba after 1945. This suggests either that the effects of the miracle drugs and residual insecticides were more pronounced outside Havana, or that there were divergent trends of age-specific mortality rates from cardiovascular diseases in the two areas.

Since nearly 60 percent of the decline in mortality from cardiovascular diseases in Havana occurred after 1931, most of it can be attributed to the availability of modern drugs. The earlier decline, betwen 1919 and 1931, was probably associated with improvements in living levels. The rest of the country appears to have followed the same developments in cardiovascular mortality as observed for Havana. The steepness of the curves in figure 11 since at least 1942, if not 1937 (for Cuba), probably indicates the effectiveness of the sulfonamides and antibiotics in reducing mortality from many other causes.

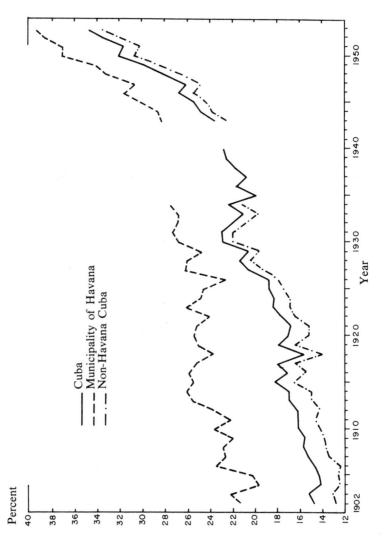

Figure 11. Deaths Attributed to Cardiovascular Diseases

Influenza, Pneumonia, and Bronchitis

These diseases, frequently associated with other causes of death, have been effectively treated only since the advent of modern drugs, specifically sulfonamides and antibiotics.[47] The influenza viruses are known to undergo changes from time to time in their antigenic components.[48] A particularly virulent strain is believed to have caused the severe pandemic of 1918. Bronchitis may be either acute or chronic. Many factors are known to be involved in its development, such as susceptibility, atmospheric pollution, and smoking.[49] Since smoking and atmospheric pollution have been on the increase during this century, McKeown, Record, and Turner concluded that reduced exposure to aetiological influences could hardly have been a factor in the declines in mortality from these diseases in England and Wales.[50] They postulated improvements in living conditions—specifically nutrition—as likely factors, and noted that, although infection rates may not have changed over time, the resistance of the host may have increased, thus leading to a reduction in the case-fatality rate.[51]

These diseases contributed 9 to 10 percent of the total mortality decline of Havana from 1901 to 1953. Only minor changes in the mortality levels from these diseases had occurred by 1931, and these appeared mainly after 1919. Between 1931 and 1943 the mortality rates from influenza, pneumonia, and bronchitis declined by about 20 percent, and over 50 percent of their total decline after 1901 was recorded between 1943 and 1953. These findings for Havana agree closely with the medical evidence and suggest that the declines from these diseases resulted mainly from the introduction of modern drugs.

The patterns in the percentages of registered deaths ascribed to influenza, pneumonia, and bronchitis shown in figure 12 indicate that, prior to the modern drugs, the share of all deaths attributed to these diseases remained fairly stationary. The wide oscillations in the curves were associated with occasional changes in the virulence of influenza. The most noticeable peak occurred in 1918, during the world-wide pandemic. The percentages of deaths ascribed to these diseases started to decline before 1945, after the appearance of sulfonamides. The higher percentages of deaths from these diseases outside Havana, compared to in the city, correspond to the difference in age distribution of population. For these particular diseases, infancy and early childhood are the times when death is most likely to occur.[52]

Diarrhea, Gastritis, and Enteritis

The gastrointestinal diseases affect primarily infants and children and are associated with poor environmental sanitation and the weaning of babies. In the early months of life, the risk of death from these diseases is small among breast-

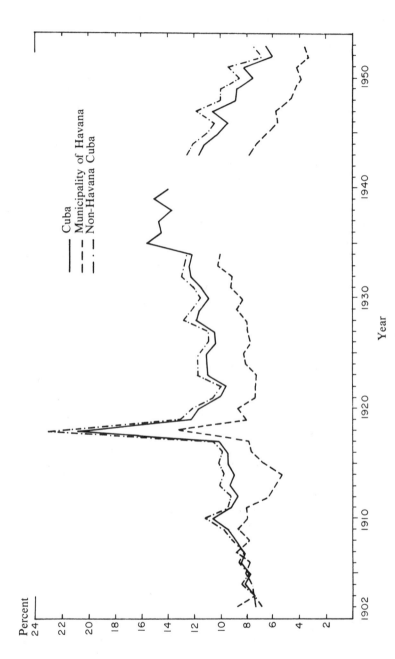

Figure 12. Deaths Attributed to Influenza, Pneumonia, and Bronchitis

fed children, but increases progressively with age, as other sources of milk are introduced or nutrition is supplemented with solid foods. With the intake of supplementary foods, the child is exposed to a gamut of common bacteria to which the body has to adapt. Where poor sanitation prevails, the bacteria counts are excessively high and produce a violent reaction in the child's system. Fluid and electrolytic imbalances result that can precipitate death or, by lowering natural defenses, lead to death from other diseases. The nutritional state is closely related to gastrointestinal mortality. The lower socioeconomic classes, which have lower protein intakes, experience not only a higher incidence of gastroenteritis but also higher mortality from these diseases than do the higher socioeconomic classes.[53]

M. W. Beaver has suggested that the decline of gastrointestinal mortality in today's developed countries has largely resulted from (aside from general improvements in sanitation) the pasteurization of milk and the growing use of canned and dried milk.[54] However, an increasing amount of evidence from developing countries, where sanitary standards are poor, indicates that increased reliance on substitutes for breast milk may have a detrimental effect on gastrointestinal mortality in young children. It has been found that a lack of elementary knowledge regarding sanitation tends to cancel out the potential benefits of milk substitutes, for example, the failure to boil water with which the milk substitutes are diluted.[55]

Housing improvements and water purification are two of the environmental advances most capable of reducing gastrointestinal mortality. However, education in personal hygiene is thought to be one of the principal keys to controlling these diseases.

The decline of mortality from diarrhea, gastritis, and enteritis in Havana from 1901 to 1953 accounted for the largest percentage decline in the total death rate—21.5 percent (see tables 14 and 15). The decline in the age-sex-standardized rates was very abrupt between 1901 and 1907. In this brief interval, it is estimated that mortality from these diseases was cut almost in half. After 1907 the decline continued at a gradual pace (with the exception of a minor upturn in 1919). Most of the decline during the first three decades of the twentieth century resulted from the extensive sanitary reforms instituted in Havana shortly after the beginning of the century, especially the efforts of the public health authorities to improve the quality and quantity of water supplies and to educate the population in proper infant care.

The considerable increase in literacy during the first decades of the century was an additional factor in the decline of mortality from gastroenteritis. The increase in literacy and the effectiveness of the health-education campaign were probably greater in Havana than in the rest of the country.

Still another cause of the decline in mortality from diarrhea, gastritis, and

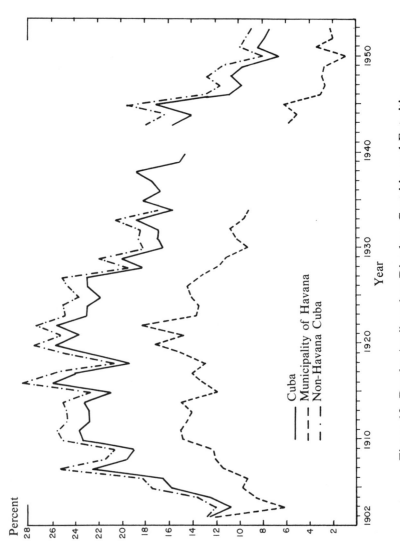

Figure 13. Deaths Attributed to Diarrhea, Gastritis, and Enteritis

enteritis may have been improved nutrition, especially in Havana. The per capita consumption of canned and dry milk in the country as a whole more than tripled during the first two decades of the century.[56] Almost all of these goods were imported and, in all likelihood, their consumption was confined mostly to the city, where higher standards of sanitation may have tended to reduce the ill effects of mother's-milk substitutes.

We can trace practically all of the improvements in sanitation and nutrition back to the early growth of the economy: improvements in sanitation resulted from an increase in government revenues, and those in nutrition (canned and dry milk), from the availability of foreign exchange with which to purchase goods abroad.

The trends in percentages of total registered deaths ascribed to diarrhea, gastritis, and enteritis shown in figure 13 imply that what occurred in Havana was only fragmentarily duplicated in the rest of the country. Nevertheless, the declines in gastroenteritis mortality probably accounted for the greatest share of the total decline in non-Havana Cuba, as in Havana. Particularly interesting in figure 13 is the substantial decline in the percentages after 1927, the year when the country began to suffer the adverse economic conditions associated with the depression of the late 1920s and early 1930s. This decline must have resulted from a drop in fertility, since it is at about this time that O. Andrew Collver estimated the earliest declines in the Cuban birth rate.[57]

After 1927, except for brief periods, the percentages of deaths attributed to diarrhea, gastritis, and enteritis continued to decline. Such a pattern suggests that the rate of mortality from these causes, as well as their proportionate share in all deaths, was on the decline, especially if we recall that mortality from many other causes was also declining. The very large gaps between the percentages of mortality from these diseases in Havana and in the rest of Cuba were probably due partly to differences in fertility and population age structure, but mainly to differences in sanitary conditions.

Certain Degenerative Diseases

This heading includes four rather diverse diseases: diabetes, nephritis, ulcers of the stomach and duodenum, and cirrhosis of the liver. This grouping was decided upon by Preston and his associates because "all [these diseases] are characterized by a sharply upward-sloping age curve of mortality."[58] These diseases, with the exception of nephritis, gained in relative importance as contributors to the total death rate as mortality declined. Since nephritis normally results from complications of bacterial infection, deaths from this cause may have declined largely for the same reasons as did deaths from other infectious diseases.

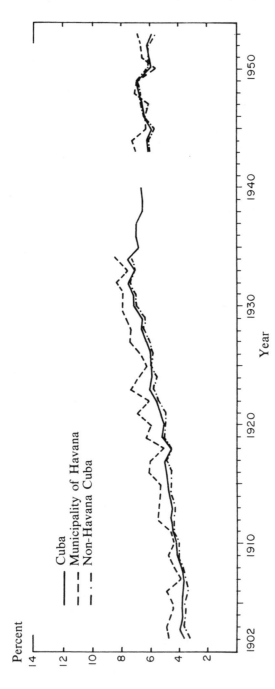

Figure 14. Deaths Attributed to Certain Degenerative Diseases

The age-sex-standardized specific death rates for these diseases in Havana show that close to 4 percent of the overall mortality decline from 1901 to 1953 was produced by reductions in this group. Only minor changes in the rates had occurred by 1931, but after that time, mortality from these diseases began to decline at a fast pace and gained momentum after 1943. The timing of the trend suggests that the decline in mortality from degenerative diseases resulted primarily from the introduction of the modern drugs after the mid-1930s. A number of these drugs are very effective against many of the infections that lead to chronic and acute nephritis, for example. In addition, a radical change in the assignment of nephritis-related causes in dealing with multiple causes of death accounted for some of the large decline in nephritis mortality by 1953.[59] The largest proportion of the deaths no longer attributed to these causes found its way into the cardiovascular diseases category.

The percentages of total deaths attributed to certain degenerative diseases, shown in figure 14, depicted a gradual tendency to increase over time up to the early 1930s, both in Havana and in non-Havana Cuba. The reversal of this trend since then reflects the impact of modern drugs. The fact that the percentages of total deaths attributed to certain degenerative diseases were higher in Havana than in non-Havana Cuba may be a result of the older age structure of the city's population.

Complications of Pregnancy

In Havana declines in mortality from complications of pregnancy contributed about 1 percent to the total mortality decline from 1901 to 1953. During the first two decades of the century, the rates of maternal mortality tended to increase, attaining their highest level in 1919.[60] By 1931 the maternal mortality rates had declined considerably. After 1931 the decline accelerated, to a very low level of mortality from complications of pregnancy by 1953—less than one-tenth of the level in 1901. Although the decrease in fertility was a contributing factor, medical advances were responsible for some of the decline in mortality from complications of pregnancy before 1931, and for most of the decline after that date.[61]

The data on percentages of deaths attributed to complications of pregnancy (figure 15) suggest that similar developments occurred in the rest of the country. During the 1940s and 1950s, public maternity hospitals were established in each of the provincial capitals to serve both the population of the cities and of the smaller towns and rural areas. The higher percentages of deaths attributed to puerperal conditions in non-Havana Cuba reflect fertility and sanitary differentials between the capital and the rest of the country, as well as differentials regarding the percentages of births that took

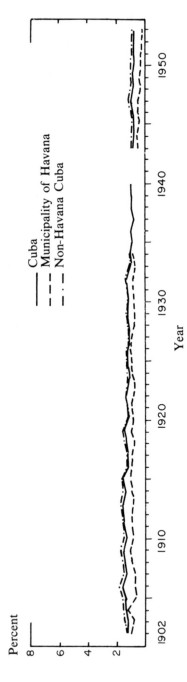

Figure 15. Deaths Attributed to Complications of Pregnancy

place in modern hospital facilities. In the case of maternal mortality, age-structure differentials between the two areas tended to minimize the differences in the percentages of deaths attributed to these causes.

Certain Diseases of Infancy

These causes of death are diverse, heavily concentrated in the first hours or days after birth, and are still difficult to diagnose properly. Thus an interpretation of secular changes in mortality from these causes is problematic, especially in Cuba, where deaths occurring within the first twenty-four hours after birth were recorded separately as stillbirths. (I excluded stillbirths from the calculation of the rates and of the estimation of the percentage distribution of deaths by cause.) It is likely that the prevalence of many of the causes of death included under "certain diseases of infancy" did not change significantly over time and, hence, that these causes' relative share of the total number of deaths increased as mortality from other causes declined. Naturally, fluctuations in fertility are likely to affect the trends in mortality from these diseases.

Some of the mortality in this group is related to endogenous causes. The intractability of these causes of death limits the potential decline in mortality from them, even in developed countries. Some of the diseases of infancy have an infectious origin; others result from injuries incurred during birth.[62] The age-sex-standardized cause-specific rates for Havana, which show an erratic pattern not observed for any other disease or group of diseases, emphasize the many uncertainties in this group. Classification problems appear to be involved in these trends.

Figure 16 shows, not unexpectedly, that the percentages of the total number of registered deaths attributed to certain diseases of infancy were higher outside of Havana than within the city. The curves reveal that the relative importance of this group of causes of death remained about the same throughout the period.

Accidents and Violence

Mortality from accidents and violence is largely independent of many of the factors that affect other causes of death, although suicides and homicides correlate with fluctuations in economic conditions in many countries. Advances in medical knowledge did have some effect, however. Improvements in surgical techniques and the use of modern drugs to combat infections resulted in the saving of many lives that otherwise would have been lost as a result of accidents and violence. An increase in automobile

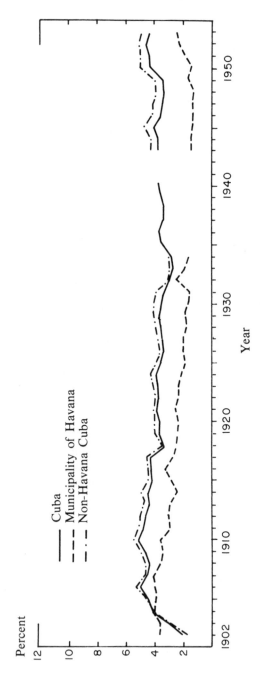

Figure 16. Deaths Attributed to Certain Diseases of Infancy

accidents tended to counteract the decline in rates of mortality from other accidents and violence.

The reduction in mortality from accidents and violence as a whole contributed between 0.5 and 1.5 percent to the mortality decline in Havana from 1901 to 1953. The highest mortality rate from these causes was in 1919 and was associated with heavy immigration in that year. Substantial declines were recorded after 1931, a year of civil unrest, and the mortality rates due to accidents and violence stabilized, with hardly any change between 1943 and 1953.

Figure 17 displays the variability in mortality from these causes from one year to the next. The curves show that as mortality from other causes was reduced, the relative importance of accidents and violence increased. The pronounced peak in the Havana curve for 1933 reflects the effects of the civil unrest that was largely confined to the city.

All Other and Unknown Causes

Reductions in mortality from causes in this category should be expected for two reasons. First, as nosological and medical concepts have improved, many of the causes included in this group have been placed in other, better-defined categories. Second, many diseases originally included in this group were of infectious origin.

The data for Havana support these interpretations. The residual group as a whole contributed about 9.5 percent to the decline of mortality in the city from 1901 to 1953. The secular trend of decline appears constant, suggesting that the removal of causes of death which became better-identifiable was a factor in the decline.

Deaths from "all other and unknown" causes accounted for a significant percentage of all deaths throughout the period, as figure 18 shows. The trends are by no means clear, but generally show that the relative importance of this group increased as deaths from previously mentioned causes declined. The large upturn observed after 1950 may correspond to the radical revision (the sixth) of the International List of Causes of Death made at that time.

Implications of the Determinants of Mortality Decline for the Evaluation of Secular Changes in Social Welfare

The preceding analysis of the determinants of mortality decline during the first half of the twentieth century provides some clues to how the process of social and economic development experienced by Cuba affected the welfare of the population. The findings strongly substantiate what the economic, educational, public expenditure, and nutritional data reviewed in Chapter 4

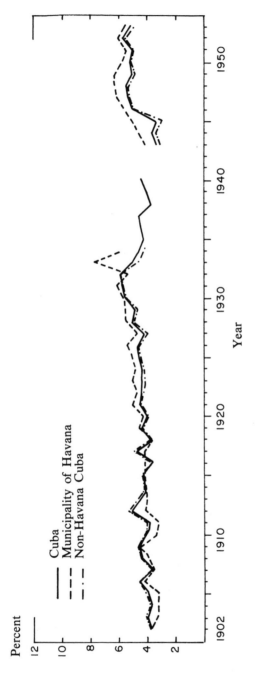

Figure 17. Deaths Attributed to Accidents and Violence

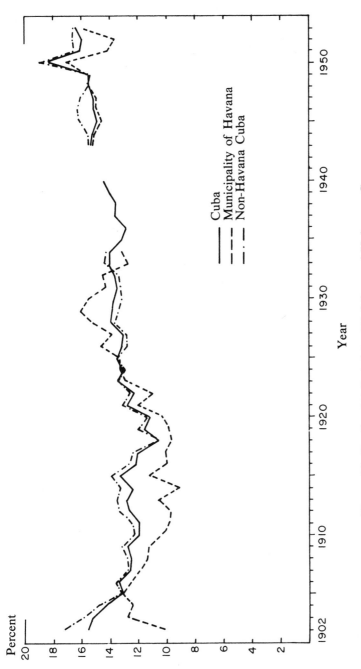

Figure 18. Deaths Attributed to All Other and Unknown Causes

suggested: that living conditions and the general welfare of the population improved considerably over most of the first three decades of the century. These data also give strong credence to the notion that, when faced with the severe economic crisis of the 1930s, living standards in Cuba deteriorated drastically, but started to improve again shortly after the Second World War.

Cuba's economic dependence on the United States was intimately tied to economic fluctuations. As Jorge Domínguez has concluded, up to about 1930, "the United States economy provided direct and indirect stimuli for substantial economic growth, while United States occupations of the island promoted public health and educational measures."[63] This same dependency was instrumental in plummeting Cuba into a period of economic chaos during the 1930s. Mortality statistics clearly reflect these changing conditions. Up to 1931, significant improvements in mortality were recorded. What is very important is that these improvements occurred at a time when medical measures were insufficient to induce drastic changes in mortality. During the first three decades of the twentieth century mortality advances were brought about largely by improvements in socioeconomic conditions and nutrition and through the provision of sanitary facilities and a wide range of public-health measures. Many of these public-health measures had gained acceptance in the more advanced countries during the 1890s, when the bacterial genesis of many diseases was demonstrated. This study has shown that those diseases that were responsible for mortality declines during the first thirty years of the century, such as tuberculosis, cardiovascular conditions, diarrhea, and many other infectious-origin diseases, reacted favorably to the increased availability of public-health measures and general improvements in sanitation, nutrition, and living conditions. In the absence of these improvements, such drastic mortality changes would not have occurred, since specific medical measures accounted for only a small proportion of the mortality declines in these decades.

During the 1930s, the trend in the decline of mortality from many diseases (tuberculosis, malaria, and others) was reversed, and at a time when every other indicator of national welfare took a turn for the worse. Of special significance is that we can directly attribute the reversals in mortality to a worsening of living conditions, since other diseases that reacted favorably to advances in medical technology continued to decline or even began to decline during the years of economic crisis. It does not seem coincidental that the 1930s were also a decade of considerable political strife, since latent tensions within the nation were undoubtedly exacerbated by the profound malaise then pervading Cuba.

The relative improvement of economic conditions in Cuba during, but especially after, the Second World War (a development reflected in the mortality statistics and in many other data sources) suggests that the welfare of the people also improved during those years. One important qualifier as far as health conditions are concerned, though, is that many of the improvements resulted from remarkable medical and chemical advances imported from abroad. These advances had a tremendous impact on mortality conditions, independent of socioeconomic changes, as the experiences of countries besides Cuba demonstrate. Yet, improved economic conditions in Cuba also contributed, since they were instrumental in the expansion of education, health services, and other areas. These improvements in the national economy were partly produced by a relatively lesser degree of dependence on conditions in foreign economies, by a greater degree of political independence, and by a lessening of the contribution of foreign trade to national income.[64]

Another very significant factor emerges from the analysis of the mortality data and is reinforced by well-known accounts of social conditions in rural Cuba during this whole period: living-condition differentials between Havana and other urban centers and rural areas, particularly the rural areas in the traditionally neglected provinces, were very substantial.[65] The health achievements in the modernized areas of the country were far greater than in the least developed. But as the data reviewed in this study reveal, even the most backward regions benefited to some extent. These benefits appear to have been particularly impressive following the appearance of the modern drugs and insecticides, the effectiveness of which is largely independent of socioeconomic conditions. The decline in malaria mortality is a case in point, since the use of DDT apparently achieved remarkable results very rapidly and at a reduced per capita cost. Other infectious diseases responded to the modern drugs and declined dramatically after the drugs began to be used throughout Cuba. Yet, by 1953, much remained to be done to bring to the rural population the health benefits present in urban areas of the country, and certainly to raise the health standards of non-Havana Cuba to the level of those in the capital.

The interpretations of the welfare of Cuba's population derived from the inspection of the mortality data agree in large part with those of the many political and economic studies dealing with the country's past. Unfortunately, these studies have not been matched by similar, detailed studies of social conditions in the country over time. In many ways we can regard the mortality statistics as a more dependable barometer of changes in social conditions than are other types of data, since we can bring a substantial amount of scientific evidence to bear when interpreting the causes for the secular behavior of the statistics.

7. The Mortality Decline in Cuba after 1953

The series of life tables for Cuba presented in Chapter 2 implies that a further improvement in mortality conditions in the country as a whole took place between 1953 and 1970. Corresponding data are not available for Havana, and the statistics we have are not adequate to define the form of the mortality trend during this period, either in Havana or in Cuba as a whole, although the data for Cuba became abundant and highly reliable by the second half of the sixties.

Although reliable measures of the trend during the late 1950s and the early 1960s are absent, it seems likely that the mortality decline may have continued at a rapid pace during that time. The national economy expanded considerably and diversified during the late 1940s and most of the 1950s.[1] Per capita income estimates showed a substantial gain between 1953 and 1958. These gains must have contributed to the continuing reduction of mortality rates.[2] Further breakthroughs in medical technology probably also contributed to declining mortality. A consistent expansion of medical facilities supported by the national health ministry and by various autonomous institutions, and the growing strength of mutualist medical associations (which provided fairly comprehensive health coverage to the urban and part of the rural population of Cuba) may have aided additional health improvements. By 1958 about half of Havana's population were members of mutualist clinics, while in other urban centers mutualist membership reached 350,000.[3] A recent estimate places Cuba's life expectancy at birth in 1960 at 64.1 years for both sexes combined. This estimate appears to confirm further substantial improvements in life expectancy after 1953.[4] If this estimate is accurate, it indicates that mortality continued to decline at a rapid rate.

Cuba probably had attained one of the most favorable mortality levels in the developing world by the end of the fifties. Some evidence suggests, however, that further and significant declines in mortality rates took place following the socialist revolution in 1959. The revolution instituted drastic changes in the social and economic structures of Cuba. These changes brought substantial improvements in living conditions to a large part of the population and placed within the reach of these groups medical advances (to which they had previously had no access) that were conducive to a considerable betterment of the overall standard of health. As a result, if the life-table measures calculated for 1970 and projected by CELADE (see Chapter 2) for later periods are near the truth, Cuba today approximates more closely the mortality conditions found in the economically advanced world than those that prevail in most other developing countries.

Some analysts have suggested that during the early years of the revolution morbidity and mortality levels—infant mortality in particular—may have increased as large numbers of physicians left the country, as social and economic disruptions took place, and as pervasive and at times severe shortages of foodstuffs and medicines occurred.[5] This interpretation may or may not be correct. It is based, though, on what I think is an insufficiently critical assessment of mortality trends at the national level, as depicted by the notoriously deficient Cuban death-register (see Appendix 1 for an evaluation of the completeness of death registration in Cuba). This interpretation depends on an analysis based on an adjusted series that obviously underestimates the actual mortality level for a time when the completeness of death registration was improving and the birth rate was rising.[6] The data available are not sufficiently trustworthy for a definite interpretation, but there is strong evidence (to be discussed) suggesting that if a worsening of health conditions did in fact occur, it was only a temporary and short-lived disturbance of the secular trend of mortality decline.

It is of particular interest that the mortality decline since the early 1960s has taken place in the absence of economic growth as measured by conventional economic indicators. During the early 1960s, economic conditions deteriorated severely.[7] Only by the mid-1960s did the economy begin to stabilize and to show limited signs of growth, or at least of a reversal of the declining trend.[8] Consequently, we can conclude that by the early 1970s, economic conditions were probably not very different from what they had been in the late 1950s, and that on a per capita basis they were probably worse, because of population growth. The Cuban economy continues to falter at the present time and, for a variety of reasons, seems incapable of entering a period of sustained growth, although there is evidence that its performance improved somewhat during the first half of the 1970s, before taking a turn for the worse by the end of the decade.

Despite the poor performance of the economy, the standard of living for the more disadvantaged social groups was upgraded. The revolutionary leadership molded an austere society by nearly eliminating the consumption of nonessential goods. It redirected national wealth toward the fulfillment of the more basic needs and thus benefited the poorest sectors of society, at the expense of high- and middle-income groups. Rural-urban differences were reduced as the state invested larger amounts of national resources in rural areas. These investments included ambitious long-range development projects designed to create an infrastructure for economic growth (such as road building, irrigation projects, and reforestation), and to create employment opportunities for the rural population and the urban unemployed.

These policies, and a commitment to full or nearly full employment, have resulted in the virtual disappearance of open unemployment (although recent evidence suggests that open unemployment may be reappearing in the Cuban economy), but largely at the expense of an efficient economy. It appears that widespread, disguised unemployment characterizes the Cuban economy, and low labor-productivity may go a long way toward explaining the economy's poor performance. Full employment at low levels of productivity serves a social function, however, since it guarantees that all members of society at least have access to the same services to satisfy basic needs.

Other development programs geared to the elimination of social and rural-urban differentials have included a literacy and general education program,[9] the provision of adequate medical services to all of the population, and various measures to upgrade housing conditions. The efforts to upgrade housing have been geared to rural areas especially, although there is evidence that only limited progress has been made and that in urban areas housing standards have deteriorated. The country as a whole faces a severe housing deficit.[10]

It is possible partly to account for the mortality changes that have occurred in Cuba over the past two decades by evaluating how these income and resource redistribution programs have affected living conditions for the less-privileged sectors of Cuban society. This study focuses attention on the extent to which these programs have expanded the coverage of public health and medical services and on the impact of increased availability of services on health conditions and mortality.

Public Health Policies

According to official sources, Cuban authorities identified four basic mechanisms in the late fifties and early sixties through which overall health standards could be raised: (1) increased emphasis on preventive medicine; (2) improvements in sanitation and related areas; (3) raising of nutritional levels for the disadvantaged social groups; and (4) education of the public regarding health matters.[11] To some degree these mechanisms implied more equitable access to the country's resources, either through wider coverage by health and other social services, or through the reduction of differentials in access to basic necessities. To a large extent, the objectives of these mechanisms were complementary and more often than not built on redistributive policies with goals extending beyond that of simply improving public health. We can evaluate the extent to which these policies may have influenced the mortality decline by reviewing some of the public-health developments that have occurred in Cuba since the revolution.

Preventive Medicine

To operate successfully, a system of preventive medicine must meet a series of fundamental requirements. These include, among others, the wide availability of medical services, and the provision of these services at no cost, or at a cost low enough to make them accessible to all socioeconomic strata of the population.

The decentralization of the medical establishment, the restructuring of medical and public-health services, and an increase in the number of public-health personnel at all levels of training have met the first requirement. In Cuba, as in many other countries, medical services had been highly concentrated in the capital and still are, to some extent.[12] Table 19 illustrates the changes in the regional distribution of medical facilities. The overall ratio of beds-to-inhabitants increased by about 13 percent during the 1958 to 1973 interval. The traditionally neglected provinces of Camagüey and Oriente recorded some of the greatest gains. In these two provinces the absolute number of hospital beds more than doubled, and the ratios of beds-to-inhabitants increased substantially. In 1958, 61.7 percent of all the hospital beds in the country were in the Province of Havana; in 1973, only 44.4 percent were found there.

Moreover, the redistribution of medical facilities has gone far beyond what table 19 indicates. Before the revolution, modern and effective medical services outside the City of Havana had been limited largely to the provincial capitals and to other large towns, although, as noted earlier, in each municipality some medical services were available. In many of the municipalities, however, these medical services did not reach much of the rural population. Beginning in the early 1960s, rural medical facilities, which provided a minimum of basic care, had been established throughout the country. By 1975 fifty-six rural hospitals had been built in the least-accessible regions of Cuba (many in mountainous areas).[13] These rural hospitals, and regional polyclinics in other areas, serve the needs of the surrounding population and as local branches to the main regional

Table 19
Regional Distribution of Hospital Beds

Province	1958		1973	
	Number of Beds	Beds per 1000 Population	Number of Beds	Beds per 1000 Population
Pinar del Río	941	2.2	1,739	3.0
Havana	17,616	9.6	18,199	7.7
Matanzas	973	2.5	2,065	3.9
Las Villas	2,917	2.7	4,920	3.5
Camagüey	1,682	2.6	4,324	4.6
Oriente	4,407	1.9	9,772	3.0
Total	28,536	4.2	41,019	4.6

Source: Ministerio de Salud Pública, *Cuba: Organización de los servicios y nivel de salud* (Havana, 1974), p. 38.

hospitals, located in the provincial capitals.

Two features built into the training of physicians and supporting staff account for the accomplishments of the rural medical programs. One of these is the requirement that newly graduated physicians serve for a specified period in a rural area. They are asigned to an area according to need, and generally serve in the more-remote locations. More-senior physicians from the regional centers provide support by periodically visiting the rural facilities.[14]

The other important feature is the multiplication of training centers for other health personnel. Many of these training centers have been located in the areas from which the students come. The assumption behind the proliferation of local training centers is that the medical needs in each area can best be served by trainees who can identify with the conditions in their communities. This policy also contributes to the reduction of the gaps between the larger cities and the rest of the country by decentralizing the location of teaching institutions.

The nationalization of medicine has satisfied the second requirement, that medical services be available to the population at low cost. The private practice of medicine has almost completely disappeared from Cuba. Most physicians today are employees of the state, although a reduced number of older physicians still practice privately. The state pays for medical and hospital services; no direct charges are made to the public.

Sanitation

Numerous efforts have been made over the years to improve the standards of hygiene and sanitation. In 1953 about 55 percent of the urban population obtained its water supply from aqueducts, but by the early 1970s, this figure had increased to 90 percent. We cannot determine the extent of these improvements before 1959, however. The number of urban centers (over one thousand population) with aqueducts increased from 175 in 1959, to 480 in 1971. At present, 98 percent of the water provided by aqueducts is chemically treated, whereas in 1959, only 21 percent of the water was similarly treated.[15] Country-wide, however, the improvements have not been as substantial. The overall percentage of dwellings receiving water from aqueducts only rose from 35.2 percent in 1953, to 40.9 percent in 1970.[16] Likewise, only relatively modest gains were made in the provision of sanitary facilities (see table 20).

Table 20
Distribution of Sanitary Facilities
(Percentages)

Year	Type of Facility				
	For Exclusive Use		For Common Use		No Facility
	Inside dwelling	Outside dwelling	Inside dwelling	Outside dwelling	
1953	31.3	29.8	—	15.7	23.2
1970	36.3	31.0	2.1	12.8	17.8

Source: Junta Central de Planificación, *La situación de la vivienda en Cuba en 1970 y su evolución perspectiva* (Havana: Editorial ORBE, 1976), p. 51

Note: A dash signifies no data available.

The excessively high costs of providing sewerage facilities and safe water to isolated rural dwellings have impeded progress in rural areas. As a result, a policy has been devised under which the rural population is encouraged to settle in small villages of about 250 families where new, modern housing, piped water, sewage disposal, schools, and medical services are provided.[17] Many of these modern rural communities have been created, although the latest figures (circa 1978) suggest that only about 5 percent of the rural population presently resides in them.

Other sanitation initiatives have been directed to the destruction of disease vectors, for example, water purification and extensive campaigns to destroy malaria-carrying mosquitoes and other carriers of disease.[18] In 1973 the World Health Organization declared Cuba a country where malaria had been eradicated.[19]

Nutrition

The Cuban government claims that improvements in nutrition have been the subject of attention, but there is some controversy as to whether or not the average nutritional status of the population has improved. Some observers suggest that, in fact, nutritional levels may have seriously deteriorated. During the early 1960s, the government introduced a system of food rationing that may have reflected a reduction in food supplies. The Cuban government stated that food rationing was necessary because of a surge in demand as the initial impact of the policies of income redistribution was felt. Other sources claimed that the food shortages resulted from economic inefficiency and a drop in agricultural productivity as the economy was socialized.[20] The rationing system is still in effect. According to official sources, the allocation system provides 2,650 calories per day to each inhabitant of Cuba, although many observers would dispute this claim, since acute shortages of some basic staples persist.[21]

There has probably been a reduction in the quality and variety of food available to middle- and upper-income groups, accompanied by some improvements in food availability for the lower socioeconomic groups. The government claims that the rationing guidelines provide for supplementary allowances to the most vulnerable population subgroups, such as children and the elderly.[22] A number of recent nutritional surveys suggest that caloric intakes are adequate, although certain vitamin deficiencies exist.[23]

Education of the Public regarding Health

The considerable reduction of illiteracy in Cuba and the upgrading of the education levels of much of the population have served as vehicles for vigorous public-health campaigns. The effective use of the printed and electronic media (all government-controlled) has been called for to aid in mass vaccination efforts (for diphtheria, poliomyelitis, whooping cough, tuberculosis, tetanus) and in popularization of knowledge of sanitation measures. Highly structured mass organizations have also been relied on to help educate all of the population concerning sanitation measures, as well as to guarantee full participation in public health.[24] The totalitarian nature of the regime has facilitated the implementation of some of these measures.

We can assess the positive effects of the measures discussed above on the health of the Cuban people by relying on diverse sources of evidence. Table 21 shows the effect of expanded medical facilities on the percentages of births taking place in medical institutions. From 1966 to 1973 the percentage of all births occurring in hospitals increased from 77.1 percent to 98.0 percent.

Table 21
Births and Maternal and Perinatal Mortality Rates in Hospitals

Year	% Births in Hospitals	· Maternal Mortality Rate[a]	Perinatal Mortality Rate[b]
1962	—	117.9	—
1963	—	113.0	—
1964	—	109.7	—
1965	—	106.9	—
1966	77.1	90.9	—
1967	79.1	90.1	—
1968	86.4	84.7	33.4
1969	92.3	86.1	33.2
1970	89.7	71.5	32.1
1971	95.6	63.9	31.4
1972	97.6	52.0	28.8
1973	98.0	54.4	28.7

Source: Ministerio de Salud Pública, *Cuba: Organización de los servicios y nivel de salud* (Havana, 1974), pp. 80, 84, and 85.

[a] per 100,000 live births.

[b] per 1,000 live births.

Note: A dash indicates no data available.

Substantial declines in maternal and perinatal mortality were associated with this trend. The increased availability of medical facilities and personnel and the considerable attention directed toward reducing infant mortality have produced notable results. The infant mortality rate was reduced from 46.7 per thousand in 1969, to 24.8 in 1977.[25] By 1979 it had declined to 19.4, and there was evidence that regional (urban-rural) differentials in infant mortality had been largely eliminated.[26] These factors and others, such as improvements in pediatric care, priority attention to high-risk pregnancies, and "widespread, free access to fertility regulations, both legal abortion and contraceptive services," have contributed to a reduction in infant and maternal mortality.[27] We can attribute this partly to the fact that the prevalence of abortion removes high-risk babies (such as the fetuses of women with many children, or women who are too young or too old) from the universe of the newborn exposed to the risk of dying.

Other evidence (see table 22) suggests that the 1953 mortality differential between the City of Havana and the rest of the country had been considerably reduced by 1970. In that year the Cuban province with the lowest estimated life expectancy was only slightly below the national average, while the Province of Havana itself, heavily influenced by the mortality experience of the capital city, had a life expectancy almost identical to the national estimate.[28] We should note, however, that the actual life expectancy for the Province of Havana was higher than the figures suggest, since many nonresidents who came to the province seeking the superior and specialized medical facilities of the capital died there. This situation contrasts with that observed in 1953, when life expectancy levels in Havana were significantly higher than for Cuba as a whole, although the life expectancy then for Havana was probably even higher than the estimate shows because of the recording of deaths of nonresidents.

Table 22
Life Expectancies at Birth

Area	Life Expectancy	
	1953	1970
Municipality of Havana	62.7[a]	—
Province of Havana		70.6[c]
Pinar del Río Province		71.0[c]
Matanzas Province		71.6[c]
Las Villas Province		71.8[c]
Camagüey Province		68.8[c]
Oriente Province		69.4[c]
Cuba	58.8[b]	70.2[d]

Sources: [a] This study, Chapter 2.

[b] Fernando González Q. and Jorge Debasa, *Cuba: Evaluación y ajuste del censo de 1953 y las estadísticas de nacimientos y defunciones entre 1943 y 1958. Tabla de mortalidad por sexo, 1952-1954,* series C, no. 124 (Santiago, Chile: Centro Latinoamericano de Demografía, 1970).

[c] Junta Central de Planificación, *Cifras sobre la niñez y la juventud cubanas* (Havana, September 1975).

[d] Junta Central de Planificación, *La esperanza o expectativa de vida* (Havana, 1974).

Note: Life expectancy rates are simple arithmetic averages for males and females.

The decline in mortality from the diarrheal diseases also illustrates how productive some of these measures have been. Stein and Susser reported in

1972 that mortality from these causes had declined considerably in Cuba, yet, paradoxically, diarrheal morbidity had not. Cuban health authorities attributed this anomaly to the fact that reporting of morbidity had improved over time. Stein and Susser, on the other hand, believed that in Cuba nutrition and medical care had improved a great deal more than had hygiene and sanitation, a conclusion confirmed by some of the data presented earlier. These authors concluded that the decline in mortality from diarrheal diseases had been achieved by rapid and effective medical intervention when the disease appear.[29] The greater availability of modern medical services and the rural population's increased awareness of the causes and cures of these diseases account for the significant decline in mortality from these afflictions, even in the presence of still-high morbidity (or infection) rates.

Since there are no comparable series of death statistics for the periods before and after the revolution, it is not easy to evaluate fully the impact of the revolution's economic and social reforms on the course of mortality decline. Separate data are not available for Havana for this period, and the gradual increase in the completeness of death registration in the rest of the country after 1959 distorts the recorded trend of the death rate in Cuba as a whole. However, we can get a perspective on the progress of Cuba's mortality transition by comparing the country's cause-specific mortality data with similar data from other nations in the Western Hemisphere. Table 23 gives the age-standardized cause-specific death rates (for selected causes) for Cuba and seven other American nations for 1970, and the age-standardized death rates for all causes combined for these same nations for circa 1970 and in 1975.[30] The age-standardized death rate for all causes in Cuba is lower than that of any other Latin American country included in the table and lies at about the same level as that of the United States at both dates.[31] The cause-specific death rates for the communicable and infectious diseases are substantially lower in Cuba than in all of the other countries shown, except Uruguay and the United States. For the degenerative diseases, Cuba occupies a middle position, between the countries that experienced earlier declines in fertility and mortality (Argentina, the United States, and Uruguay) and those that have lagged behind Cuba in their demographic transition. Data on cause-specific mortality for dates around 1975 exhibit similar patterns.

We can further assess the advances that Cuba has made in reducing mortality during the last two decades by comparing the levels of life expectancy at birth estimated for Cuba in 1953 and in 1970 (the two dates for which dependable life-table estimates are available) with corresponding data from other countries (see table 24).[32] By 1953 Cuba, as noted in Chapter 2, already had a greater life expectancy than many other Latin American countries. Only countries that were most advanced economically in 1950 exceeded Cuba's life expectancy (Canada and the United States and, to a lesser extent, Argentina, Uruguay, and Puerto Rico). All of the other countries included in table 24 were either at about the same level of life expectancy as Cuba (Jamaica, Trinidad and Tobago, and Costa Rica) or markedly below. By the early 1970s, the estimated Cuban life expectancy at birth was nearly comparable to the estimates for the most advanced countries in the Americas (Canada and the United States), higher than Argentina's, in view of the differences in levels of cause-specific rates between Cuba and that country, and about two years higher than that of Uruguay and Costa Rica.[33]

Improvements in medical technology during the last two decades throughout the world have benefited every country in the area of mortality declines. Examples include the vaccine against poliomyelitis, which only began to be used extensively throughout the world in the mid- to late-1950s, and the measles vaccine, widely used even later than the polio vaccine. Also, additional progress in further reducing mortality levels was almost certainly made between 1953 and the time when the institutional reforms in Cuba were begun (1959). Therefore, had the institutional changes carried out in Cuba after the revolution not occurred, improvements in life expectancy would have come about anyway. However, it is significant that by 1970, Cuba had outpaced the post-1950 mortality declines of countries such as Argentina, Costa Rica, Jamaica, and Trinidad and Tobago, which had had life expectancies at birth similar to or higher than Cuba's. In my opinion, it is thanks to the reforms in Cuba since 1959 that the country has gained, at a minimum, two to three years more in life expectancy at birth than some of these countries. The reduction of social and regional inequalities in general and, in particular, in access to public health and health care, appears to be the main causative factor behind Cuba's impressive gain in life expectancy.[34] Some years later Costa Rica also appears to have made comparable progress in lowering mortality by reducing these inequities.

The reshaping of Cuban society has resulted in more equitable access to medical attention, food, and the general amenities of life for the whole population. We can state unequivocally that the reductions in mortality during the 1960s were determined mainly by the wide use of modern medical resources, ranging from drugs and vaccinations to the implementation of public-health technologies and the considerable expansion of medical facilities. It is very significant that these achievements were especially notable in rural areas of the country, despite the fact that sanitation facilities there were improved only to a limited extent, as the housing, water supply, and dwelling data indicate.

Table 23

Cause-Specific Death Rates for Selected American Countries, circa 1970

Cause of Death*	Cause-Specific Death Rate**							
	Cuba	Argentina	Costa Rica	Chile	Panama	United States	Uruguay	Venezuela
All infective and parasitic diseases (000-136)	34.7	75.0	103.3	88.1	96.7	6.2	34.8	90.7
Enteritis and other diarrheal diseases (008-009)	14.3	31.4	55.1	42.0	33.5	1.2	13.6	44.0
Tuberculosis, all forms (010-019)	3.8	11.1	7.5	21.3	15.9	1.2	5.0	10.4
Malignant neoplasms (140-209)	76.5	90.7	73.4	85.9	46.4	77.1	101.2	61.2
Malignant neoplasm of trachea, bronchus, or lung (162)	16.7	15.2	4.1	6.2	3.7	15.3	13.5	6.1
Diseases of the heart (390-429)	102.6	129.8	86.8	87.1	71.6	147.5	110.0	90.6
Cerebrovascular diseases (430-438)	40.5	48.8	30.1	50.3	34.5	38.8	56.9	32.9
Influenza and pneumonia (470-474, 480-486)	31.7	45.5	52.6	123.6	43.4	17.1	23.2	44.6
Complications of pregnancy (630-678)	3.5	6.1	6.0	8.2	8.7	0.7	3.0	7.5
Symptoms and ill-defined conditions (780-796)	3.2	56.4	62.4	46.2	107.3	8.9	38.9	146.2

Table 23—*Continued*

Cause of Death*	Cause-Specific Death Rate**							
	Cuba	Argentina	Costa Rica	Chile	Panama	United States	Uruguay	Venezuela
All accidents (E800-E949, E980-E989)	32.4	46.9	40.6	81.4	42.6	48.9	35.4	51.7
Suicide (E950-E959)	12.2	7.7	3.4	5.4	2.4	8.6	7.3	6.5
Age-standardized death rate (All causes combined)***								
1970	4.8	7.1	6.3	8.1	5.9	4.8	5.9	6.9
1975	4.3	N.A.	5.0	6.5	5.5	4.4	6.1	6.5

Sources: Pan American Health Organization (WHO), *Health Conditions in the Americas, 1969-1972* (Washington, D.C., 1974), pp. 130-173; and idem, *Health Conditions in the Americas, 1973-1976* (Washington, D.C., 1978), pp. 138-165.

* Causes of death are grouped according to the Eighth Revision of the International List of Causes of Death.

** Cause-specific rates are shown per 100,000 population, for both sexes combined. They have been standardized to the Latin American population age distribution.

*** The age-standardized death rate for all causes combined is per 1,000 population and has been standardized to the age distribution of the population of Latin America.

N.A. means no data available.

Table 24
Estimated Life Expectancies at Birth for Selected Western Hemisphere Nations

Country		Life Expectancy at Birth		
Cuba	(1953)	58.8[a]	(1970)	70.2[d]
Argentina	(1947)	60.1	(1970)	65.7
Canada	(1951)	68.6	(1972)	72.7
Chile	(1952)	*50.2*	(1972)	62.8
Colombia	(1951)	*49.2*	(1973)	59.0
Costa Rica	(1950)	*55.5*	(1972)	67.8
Ecuador	(1950)	*47.9*	(1965-70)	61.0
El Salvador	(1950)	*47.2*	(1969-72)	55.0
Guatemala	(1950)	*40.7*	(1971)	52.4
Jamaica	(1953)	59.1	(1971)	66.7
Mexico	(1950)	*47.6*	(1969-71)	60.0
Panama	(1950)	*50.2*	(1969-71)	65.0
Peru	(1961)	*48.9*[b]	(1970-75)	55.0
Puerto Rico	(1955)	67.8[c]	(1970)	72.1[c]
Trinidad and Tobago	(1946)	54.1	(1971)	66.6
United States	(1950)	68.3	(1971)	71.4
Uruguay	(1950)	68.8	(1971)	68.1
Venezuela	(1950)	52.6	(1971)	65.0

Sources: Except as noted, Pan American Health Organization (WHO), *Health Conditions in the Americas; 1969-1972* (Washington D.C., 1974), p. 13; and Eduardo E. Arriaga, *New Life Tables for Latin American Populations in the Nineteenth and Twentieth Centuries*, Population Monograph Series, no. 3 (Berkeley and Los Angeles: University of California Press, 1968); and table 4 of this study. Differences between the estimates given in these sources reflect data biases not covered when accepting official figures.

Note: Values in italics have been obtained from Arriaga.

[a]Estimate by Fernando González Q. and Jorge Debasa, *Cuba: Evaluación y ajuste del censo de 1953 y las estadísticas de nacimientos y defunciones entre 1943 y 1958. Tabla de mortalidad por sexo, 1952-1954*, Centro Latinoamericano de Demografía, series C, no. 124 (Santiago, Chile, 1970).

[b] The value given by the Pan American Health Organization for 1950 is obviously erroneous. It exceeds by almost ten years the life expectancy calculated by Arriaga for 1961.

[c] The 1970 (1969-71) value from United Nations, *Demographic Yearbook, 1974* (New York, 1974), table 33, p. 1016; 1955 (1954-56) value from idem, *Demographic Yearbook, 1966* (New York, 1966), table 21, p. 570. In each case, the values for both sexes combined have been derived by averaging the figures for the two sexes.

[d] Junta Central de Planificación, *La esperanza o expectativa de vida* (Havana, 1974).

The key to the effectiveness of the reforms, therefore, was the political commitment to extend those services to all the population and to place a premium on measures that would minimize the ill effects of disease. Government decisions that affected the allocation of national resources reversed a situation in which not all sectors of society had access to or could afford these services and facilities. Public-health campaigns and significant advances in average educational levels facilitated these developments because the population became more aware of what could be done to avoid disease and, when stricken, how to take advantage of the ubiquitous medical facilities.

Particularly interesting is the fact that mortality declines took place in the upper range of life expectancies achievable at present. The additional gains in life expectancy were made possible by the reduction of infant and childhood mortality, where further mortality reductions are difficult to achieve, and in a country with relatively low per capita income and experiencing serious economic difficulties.

The assessment of factors leading to the mortality decline since the revolution would not be complete if I were to neglect a discussion of the considerable economic costs that achieving mortality declines has entailed and the means at Cuba's disposal to pay those costs. This is a significant consideration because it suggests that what Cuba has achieved could hardly be replicated in other developing countries with similarly scarce resources and competing economic needs. It seems highly unlikely that Cuba could have directed so many resources to social areas such as education and health in the absence of massive amounts of Soviet economic aid (conservatively estimated at over $8.25 billion over the 1961-1976 period).[35] The new society sponsored by the revolution, as Cole Blasier has indicated, was made possible only by this economic assistance. The reasons why the Soviet Union has been willing to underwrite the economic survival of the Cuban revolution are beyond the scope of this study but have received considerable attention from many political analysts. Unquestionably, serious disruptions produced by a drastic process of revolutionary change greatly intensified the economic problems with which revolutionary Cuba had to contend. Yet, it seems undeniable that foreign assistance on a scale not received by any other poor nation was highly instrumental, if not essential, in facilitating the progress made. It goes without saying, however, that the transformation of Cuban society was also achieved after tremendous political and social upheavals that other nations may not be willing to or capable of enduring.

For these and other reasons Cuba's experience may have only limited relevance to other poor nations, and for whatever reasons, when we consider exclusively the mortality indices analyzed in this study, it seems reasonable to conclude that the welfare of the Cuban people, overall, has improved over the last two decades. The balance sheet may not be as conclusive, however, when we consider other dimensions of well-being and some of the costs that the achievements of the Cuban revolution have entailed. The range of opinion about the Cuban revolution and about what it has represented to the Cuban people is wide indeed.

8. Summary and Conclusions

Before the twentieth century, premodern mortality conditions prevailed in Cuba. Limited statistical evidence for Havana and other parts of the country indicates that mortality was high and fluctuating, as a result of frequent and violent attacks of epidemic diseases.

Cuba took its first step in the transition to a modern regime of mortality after the end of the Spanish-American War, in 1898, when United States military forces occupied the country for nearly four years. During those years, sweeping sanitary reforms and public-health activities caused an abrupt drop in the level of mortality. The data for Havana indicate a decrease of close to 30 percent in the crude death rate in the city by 1902, in comparison with the average of earlier decades.

Table 25 compares estimates of life expectancy at birth in Cuba and Havana with those of selected countries in several parts of the world. The data indicate that the mortality conditions in Cuba at the end of the United States military occupation were more favorable than those of most other developing countries. Two exceptions are Argentina and Jamaica.[1] It appears certain that life expectancy in Cuba at that time was higher than in Brazil, Chile, Guatemala, Mexico, Sri Lanka, or Taiwan, and possibly higher than in Costa Rica. We can attribute Cuba's relative advantage to the sanitary reforms instituted under the United States military administration. However, even after those reforms, Cuba lagged some ten to twenty years behind the most advanced European countries and the United States in life expectancy at birth.

During the next two decades, up to 1919, Cuba made a further, modest gain in life expectancy. Temporary increases in mortality from influenza, smallpox, and malaria around 1919 probably disturbed the secular trend. However, the earlier gain was strengthened during this period. It is noteworthy that some of the other developing countries listed in table 25

Table 25
Trends in Life Expectancy at Birth

Place/Year	Life Expectancy at Birth	Place/Year	Life Expectancy at Birth
Cuba		Havana	
1905	36.4	1901	37.2
1915	37.2	1907	39.1
1925	39.2	1919	41.3
1937	46.4	1931	50.8
1953	58.8	1943	54.0
1970	70.2	1953	62.7
Argentina		Brazil	
1895-99	36.7	1900	29.4
1930-34	58.5	1920	32.0
1947	61.1	1940	36.7
1955-59	66.2	1950	43.0
1965-70	67.1	1960	55.5
Chile		Costa Rica	
1907	30.1	1892	30.5
1920	30.5	1927	40.0
1930	35.2	1950	55.5
1940	38.1	1963	63.6
1952	50.2	1972	67.8
1960	56.5		
1972	62.8		
Denmark		England and Wales	
1890-94	48.0	1896	46.0
1921-25	61.1	1956	70.5
1931-35	62.9	1971	72.0
1951-55	71.2		
1970-71	73.3		
Guatemala		Jamaica	
1893	23.6	1880-82	38.4
1921	25.8	1923	38.4
1940	30.4	1946	53.0
1950	40.7	1966	68.0
1964	51.3	1970	68.5
1971	52.4		
Japan		Mexico	
1899-1903	44.4	1900	25.3
1920-25	42.6	1910	27.6
1947	52.0	1921	34.7
1955	65.5	1930	33.9

Table 25—*Continued*

Place/Year	Life Expectancy at Birth	Place/Year	Life Expectancy at Birth
1968	71.7	1940	38.8
1972	73.2	1950	47.6
		1960	58.0
		1972	63.0
Norway		Sri Lanka (Ceylon)	
1891-1895	50.4	1910-12	31.4
1911-15	58.9	1920-22	33.2
1941-45	65.3	1946	42.8
1951-55	72.9	1956	59.3
1966-70	74.0	1967	65.9
Sweden		Taiwan	
1928-32	63.1	1906	28.3
1948-52	71.4	1909-11	34.0
1972	74.7	1921	36.5
		1950	55.5
		1959	66.5
		1972	69.4
United States			
1890	43.5		
1950	68.4		
1973	71.3		

Sources: Eduardo E. Arriaga, *New Life Tables for Latin American Populations in the Nineteenth and Twentieth Centuries*, Population Monograph Series, no. 3 (Berkeley and Los Angeles: University of California Press, 1968); John D. Durand, "Report of Workshop in History of the Mortality Transition," unpublished (Philadelphia: Graduate Group in Demography, Population Studies Center, University of Pennsylvania, January-May 1975), p. 22; Pan American Health Organization (WHO), *Health Conditions in the Americas, 1969-72* (Washington, D.C., 1974), p. 13; and this study.

also experienced relatively small increases in life expectancy during the first two decades of this century. Although Mexico and Taiwan did make large gains during this period, they started from lower levels and failed to achieve the level estimated for Cuba by the end of the period. For the more advanced countries, on the other hand, the 1900-1920 period was one of large reductions in mortality. In the early 1920s, Denmark, Norway, and Sweden attained life expectancy levels not reached in Cuba until the 1950s.

Between 1919 and 1931 the pace of life expectancy gains accelerated in

Cuba, although faults in the data lead to some reservations. The decade of the 1920s was likewise a period of relatively rapid gains in a number of other developing countries, notably Chile and Japan, and probably also Costa Rica, Sri Lanka, and Taiwan. Meanwhile, the pace of gains in life expectancy slowed significantly in some of the more advanced countries, for example, in Denmark and Norway. Thus Cuba's disadvantage in regard to life expectancy, compared with the vanguard countries, diminished during this period.

The estimates for Havana during the 1930s and early 1940s show some deceleration of the trend of mortality decline, and the less-dependable data for Cuba as a whole suggest a similar slowdown. Nevertheless, Cuba in the early 1940s was still ahead of most other developing countries in life expectancy. Cuba, in company with Jamaica and Costa Rica, continued to occupy an intermediate position in the international array of countries by levels of life expectancy. The more-advanced European countries and the United States continued to experience relatively moderate gains in life expectancy during the 1930s.

The years following the Second World War saw a decided acceleration in the rate of mortality decline in Cuba, as in much of the rest of the less-developed world. The life expectancy estimates for Cuba and Havana show large gains between 1943 and 1953. Other developing countries experienced extraordinarily rapid gains at about the same time. The gains in more-developed countries were generally smaller, although still sizable. In the late 1940s or early 1950s Cuba, Costa Rica, and Jamaica retained their intermediate position, between the vanguard countries and the majority of countries in the less-developed regions. Very substantial gains in life expectancy in Japan, Taiwan, and Sri Lanka also placed these countries among those in intermediate positions.

Even though the size of Cuba's gain between 1953 and 1970 (in absolute number of years) was smaller than the gains of most other developing countries listed in table 25, the significance of Cuba's gain was equal to or greater than the other countries' gains because of the difficulty of achieving further gains at high levels of life expectancy.

The general pattern of the secular trend of life expectancy in Cuba fits the three-phased mortality transition model postulated by John Durand.[2] During the first phase, slow gains in life expectancy are recorded. Frequently, these gains are wiped out by unpredictable reversals of the trend. A second phase follows in which the earlier gains are strengthened and a significant acceleration in the growth rate of life expectancy is achieved. Finally, as the mortality transition is completed—as the ceiling of attainable life expectancy is approached—gains in life expectancy become very slow and small.

After the large initial decline of mortality, during the years of the United States military occupation, Cuba remained for about two decades in phase 1 of the transition, that is, a period in which mortality declined at a slow and irregular pace. Around 1920 the trend shifted into phase 2, when rapid gains in life expectancy began. Probably sometime in the late 1960s, Cuba reached phase 3 of its mortality transition, when it attained a life expectancy level comparable to those found in more-developed countries. It seems unlikely that further large gains will occur in the foreseeable future. A peculiarity of the Cuban case, probably duplicated in Chile, is that after the beginning of phase 2, a period (from 1931 to 1943) intervened in which the rate of gain in life expectancy was temporarily slowed, probably as a result of economic difficulties. Gains resumed at a much faster tempo after the Second World War.

The decline in mortality between 1898 and 1902 can definitely be attributed to the far-ranging sanitary reforms instituted in the country while it was occupied by the United States Army. Efforts to improve sanitation were made primarily in the major urban sectors, with Havana receiving the greatest benefits. In that city, major declines were recorded in mortality from yellow fever, malaria, smallpox, diphtheria, infantile tetanus, typhoid fever, and tuberculosis.

After Cuba obtained independence in 1902, it remained under the political tutelage of the United States for decades. The incorporation in the Cuban constitution of the Platt Amendment, whereby the United States was authorized to intervene in Cuban affairs in certain circumstances, such as the failure of the Cuban government to follow through on the plans for improving the sanitation of Cuban cities, formalized the ascendancy of American interests in Cuban affairs. The United States justified the inclusion of this provision in the Platt Amendment by claiming that it was designed not only to protect the health of the Cuban people, but also to protect the American population residing in the southern ports of the United States. The Platt Amendment also provided guarantees to foreign investors (primarily from the United States), who poured over one billion dollars into the Cuban economy during the first three decades of the twentieth century. These investments and the full opening of the United States market to Cuban sugar provided a period of economic prosperity that lasted until a few years before the World Depression of the 1930s.

Although only a relatively small decline in the overall level of mortality occurred in the City of Havana between 1901 and 1919, mortality from certain infectious diseases and gastrointestinal ailments slowed considerably during that time. Children in particular benefited from these mortality declines. Further sanitation work in the city and increased consumption of dried and canned milk were probably influential in this respect. During this time the distribution of free antiseptic-packages for the care of the umbilicus of the newborn drastically reduced infant mortality from neonatorum tetanus in Havana. During these two decades, however, substantial increases in mortality from malignant and benign tumors and from cardiovascular diseases were recorded. These apparent increases were probably due at least partly to improvements in the diagnosis of cause of death, since a substantial decline occurred in the rates for the residual category, "all other and unknown causes."

Limited evidence for the rest of the country implies that similar mortality declines were occurring at a slower pace outside of Havana. The establishment of a nationwide health ministry in 1907, of governmental programs of environmental sanitation and control of specific diseases, and of government-funded medical facilities, all had a role in the mortality decline during these years. Privately financed mutualist societies, which provided medical services on a sort of prepayment plan, also contributed. Increasing educational levels were effective in heightening popular awareness of health hazards and knowledge of defenses against disease.

The expansion of the Cuban economy during the first two decades of this century, when demand for sugar in the world markets was growing and prices were favorable, facilitated the government's investment in the development of health facilities and infrastructure. Of course, there was a delay in the influence of such investments on the mortality trend. Their full impact was delayed, in fact, until the 1919-1931 period.

The growing supplies of foreign exchange derived from sugar exports also enabled the country to increase the imports on which it depended to a large extent for food, resulting in an apparent improvement in nutrition during this period of economic prosperity. Improved nutrition had a delayed but favorable effect on the mortality trend from 1919 to 1931, and we can see the influence of improved nutrition in the dramatic reduction of tuberculosis and cardiovascular mortality during this period.

Continuing trends of decline in mortality from infectious diseases and from gastroenteritis suggest that public-health advances, further gains in literacy, and improvements in medical practice also contributed to the mortality decline between 1919 and 1931. Growing private expenditures on medical services, through the mutualist associations, complemented governmental expenditures on health-related programs.

The deceleration in the rate of mortality decline during the 1930s and early 1940s corresponds to a period of intense economic crisis that began in Cuba even before the Great Depression abroad. The international demand for sugar was curtailed, and limitations were imposed by the United States and other foreign governments on imports of Cuban sugar. The result was a severe deterioration of the Cuban economy. Food and other imports had to be drastically reduced, and there are strong indications that severe cuts were made in many government expenditures. A large, epidemic outbreak of malaria occurred in the mid-1930s, and respiratory tuberculosis mortality reversed its downward trend.

Mortality from some causes of death did decline between 1931 and 1943, such as death associated with the puerperal state, with cardiovascular diseases, and with influenza, pneumonia, and bronchitis. These diseases were vulnerable to the sulfonamides, which were first used widely in the mid- to late-1930s.

Between 1943 and 1953 the rate of mortality decline accelerated substantially. Havana and the rest of the country recorded large declines in mortality from respiratory tuberculosis, from other infectious and parasitic diseases, from influenza, pneumonia, and bronchitis, from gastroenteritis, from certain degenerative diseases, from complications of pregnancy, and from the "other and unknown" causes. Only mortality from malignant and benign tumors increased during this period. It is apparent that the mortality declines for many causes resulted in large part from the increased use of sulfonamides, the introduction of new antibiotics after the Second World War, and, in the case of malaria, from the use of residual insecticides after 1945. A marked improvement in the economy at the time also undoubtedly aided the mortality decline.

The socialist revolution of 1959 brought about major social and economic changes in Cuba. One of the most important was the country-wide income redistribution, which reduced the great disparity in living conditions that had previously existed between the cities and rural areas. The extension of medical services to the whole country and advances in sanitation improved the health standard of Cuba dramatically after the revolution. Mass-vaccination campaigns, increased literacy, rural hospital facilities and medical services, and better nutrition for the lower socioeconomic stratum of the population were the main channels by which mortality was reduced. Gastroenteritis mortality in infants declined significantly, mainly as a result of the provision of effective medical services, although the prevalence of the disease did not diminish to the same extent. Other infectious diseases, easily controllable with present-day medical knowledge, have practically disappeared from Cuba. These developments have permitted Cuba to attain a very favorable life expectancy level, distinctly higher than the levels in most other developing countries. I estimate that the gain in life expectancy in Cuba between 1953 and 1970 exceeded by two to three years what might have taken place without the revolution.

In many respects the Cuban mortality experience was unique. Whereas mortality responded as much to social, economic, and medical developments in Cuba as it did in other countries, these influences were mediated to an unusual extent by political factors. The military occupation and following political and economic subjugation of Cuba to the United States contributed to the early growth of the economy, growth that favored an early mortality decline.[3]

However, this same dependency retarded Cuba's growth later, as the country was at the mercy of economic forces beyond its control, for example, fluctuations in the demand for sugar in the international markets and the quotas imposed on sugar imports by the United States. As a result, the country underwent an economic crisis during the 1930s that was much more severe and prolonged than that experienced by the industrialized countries. The living conditions of the Cuban people deteriorated sufficiently to cause a slowdown in the secular trend of mortality decline, if not a temporary reversal. The evidence that the government curtailed expenditures in health-related areas and that private enterprise curtailed expenditures for health services is convincing. Finally, in the late 1950s and early 1960s, another momentous political change had a great impact on the trend of mortality.

Relative Impact of Different Determinants in the Cuban Mortality Decline

Given the uncertainties associated with the statistical base of this study and the tentative nature of the interpretation of the determinants of the mortality decline, it is difficult to establish with confidence the relative importance of different factors in Cuba's mortality transition. We can make a preliminary assessment, however, by focusing on the distinct transition stages that, with some confidence, we can identify, and by summarizing within each stage those factors that appear to have been most influential (table 26).

In a broad sense we can separate the factors responsible for the mortality decline within each stage into two distinct groups: mediating mechanisms and direct mechanisms. We may refer to the two most important mediating mechanisms as political will and economic conditions. The first, political will, was a crucial mediating factor during both the early and late stages of the mortality decline. In both stages this mediating mechanism made possible the implementation of profound reforms, although of differing natures. The United States military government had the will, technical knowledge, and resources to revolutionize Cuban sanitary and public-health

Table 26
Stages and Determinants of Cuba's Mortality Transition

Period	Stage	Estimated Gain in Life Expectancy	Determinants
1898-1902	Sudden and rapid onset of mortality decline	4-5 years	Political will as paramount mediating mechanism and instrumental in implementation of sweeping sanitary and public-health reforms, including widespread use of then-known mortality-reducing preventive means. Financial resources of government important facilitator of reforms. Little part played by improvements in socioeconomic conditions or nutrition, because of rapidity of change. War devastated country, but reforms significant enough to reduce mortality levels well below peacetime levels.
1902-1919	Consolidation	4-5 years	Improved economic conditions were important mediating factors. Continued expansion of sanitary and public-health measures and facilities. Nutrition and significant advances in education began to play an important role.
1919-1931	Accelerated mortality decline	7-8 years	Influenced by improvements in socioeconomic conditions operating with some time lag. Improvements in nutrition and further educational improvements critical. Expansion of public-health measures, sanitary facilities, medical services promoted better awareness of disease prevention and served as mechanisms to curtail spread of disease.
1931-1943	Stagnation in trend of declining mortality	5-6 years	Largely induced by drastic deterioration in economic conditions. Nutritional standards of sanitary facilities reduced. Expansion of sanitary facilities at a standstill during early part of period. Medical breakthroughs that operated independently of economic conditions responsible for some of most noticeable declines toward end of period.

Table 26—*Continued*

Period	Stage	Estimated Gain in Life Expectancy	Determinants
1943-1958	Very rapid mortality decline	11-12 years	Produced by unprecedented break-throughs in medical and chemical technology. Improved economic conditions and nutrition, and expanded medical facilities possible contributors.
1959-1980	Completion of mortality transition	8-9 years	Political will instrumental in making modern medical and public-health measures for prevention and cure of disease accessible to all of population. Considerable educational achievements and improved nutrition for more-disadvantaged social groups facilitated somewhat completion of stage. Services capable of counteracting potentially negative effects of deteriorated economy expanded. Foreign economic assistance permitted diversion of scarce resources to social areas.

Source: This study.

standards. Some six decades later, the Cuban revolution completely revamped the socioeconomic structures of the nation. One consequence was a process of redistribution that placed within the reach of the formerly more-marginalized sectors of Cuban society modern medical and public-health resources to which they had had no access.

The second mediating mechanism, economic conditions, was very significant over the first four decades of the century. To a large extent, it determined the extent of and rate at which mortality declines were achieved, since the growth of the economy affected how the direct mechanisms influencing mortality changes operated. In times of economic prosperity, mortality declined; in less-prosperous times, mortality declined less. The importance of economic conditions as a determinant of mortality declines lessened sometime during the late 1930s. We may even argue that since 1959, the role of economic conditions as a determinant of the mortality decline became almost negligible. Other economic considerations, such as distribution of wealth, became more important. Equalized access to the nation's resources was a key ingredient in the mortality decline. Earlier inequalities had obviously hindered the achievement of more-substantial gains in life expectancy.

We can estimate the relative importance of the direct mechanisms in the overall mortality decline by first considering how important they might have been within each of the stages defined in table 26, and second, by making rough estimates of the magnitude of the overall mortality decline within each stage. The latter is far from simple, since, as I have discussed in this study (and in the technical appendices), biases in the Havana and Cuba life tables do not permit a sufficiently rigorous establishment of the tempo of the mortality decline. This is especially true for the first four decades of the century. I derived my rough estimate of the gains in life expectancy in each of the stages from an assessment of the Havana and Cuba evidence, from other available evidence (cited at various points of this study), and from the nature of the estimating biases. These estimates assume a forty-two-year gain in life expectancy at birth for both sexes combined, from 1898 to 1980, that is, from an average life expectancy at birth of thirty years before the first public-health and sanitary reforms, during the 1898-1902 period, to the present estimated life expectancy of seventy-two years.[4]

We can attribute practically all of the gains during the first stage (1898-1902) to public-health and sanitary reforms imported into the country. Smallpox vaccination—a broadly defined medical measure—made a small contribution as did perhaps (but only to a limited extent) improvements in nutrition.

From 1902 to 1931 improved economic conditions facilitated the implementation and expansion of public-health and sanitary measures because resources were available for the construction and improvement of sanitation and infrastructural facilities (such as water distribution systems and paved streets), for the wide distribution of known preventive measures for specific diseases, and for environmental sanitation. All of these measures were conducive to the avoidance of communicable diseases, and were aided to a significant degree by considerable improvements in educational standards and by public-health education campaigns that made the better-educated population more aware of disease prevention. Nutrition improvements during this period, especially among the lower socioeconomic groups, had an equally important effect, as considerable declines in causes of death highly responsive to nutritional state indicate.

By the late 1920s, and for some years thereafter, the deterioration of the national economy interrupted further progress in sanitation and led to worsened food-intake levels. Both of these factors had negative consequences for the trend of mortality decline. Yet, during this stage, particularly toward the end, mortality from some diseases began to decline or continued to decline, as the earlier, dramatic breakthroughs in medicine (such as the sulfonamides) began to exert a powerful influence on mortality trends.

The influence of medical breakthroughs on the mortality decline has been even more pronounced since the end of the Second World War. The appearance of miracle drugs (antibiotics), vaccines, and insecticides has made possible the attainment of rapid mortality declines almost independent of changes in economic conditions. These declines in mortality were accomplished, to a great extent, without major improvements in sanitation facilities and with only a limited expansion of public-health efforts. As the experience since the 1960s suggests, the full effect of modern medical advances only came to fruition when placed within the reach of all groups, even though all of the population has yet to experience the positive impact of modern sanitary facilities.

In summary, the evidence reviewed in this study suggests that over the whole period in question the main determinants of mortality changes were developments in medical and chemical means to combat disease—if amply defined—since those means have contributed to the more-substantial gains in life expectancy experienced since the late 1930s, at the earliest. Of the total estimated gain in life expectancy from 1898 to 1980, over half (some twenty-three years) has been achieved since these measures became available.

The development of chemical and medical treatment also contributed, to a lesser extent, to the earlier gains. During the earlier stages, the implementation of sanitary and public-health measures was likely to have been the most important factor, but a factor aided to an indeterminate extent by substantial educational improvements. Educational improvements were also involved in the gains during the last stage of the trend, given that those improvements facilitated the use of preventive and curative measures the importance of which was more readily grasped by a better-educated populace.

Improvements in nutrition are a final direct factor involved in the mortality decline. Particularly during the first quarter of this century, there were very significant declines in mortality from specific causes known to respond favorably to a better diet, and during the 1930s, when the average nutritional intake took a turn for the worse, there was a reversal in the declining trend of mortality for these causes.

My conclusions, derived from an examination of the Cuban experience, support the evidence mustered by Eduardo Arriaga and Kingsley Davis that indicates that the link between declining mortality and socioeconomic conditions weakened over time in Latin America, as factors exogenous to a country's socioeconomic conditions (such as imported medical treatments) gained in importance.[5] My conclusions also reinforce Preston's that mortality has not become dissociated from standards of living over time, since, as he stated, improvements in medical and sanitary knowledge permit higher life expectancy levels at lower income levels.[6] What the most recent Cuban evidence shows, however, is that conventionally used measures of welfare, such as per capita income (as Preston himself suggests), may not be the best indicators of development. Rather than an overall summary measure of development, what appears to be more important is the distribution of benefits of development.

Implications of the History of Cuban Mortality

Similarities between the mortality transition in Cuba and that of other Latin American nations studied by Eduardo Arriaga and Kingsley Davis, and the fact that a number of less-developed countries in other regions experienced an acceleration of their mortality decline at about the same time as Cuba (1920), suggest that these simultaneous developments involved some common causal influences.[7] John Durand observed that the trends of increase in life expectancy in Japan, Jamaica, Taiwan, and Sri Lanka, for example, speeded up decidedly in the 1920s.[8] The Cuban trend did so at approximately the same time, and table 25 suggests that it was the same with Chile. A monograph by Thomas Birnberg and Stephen Resnick suggests a plausible hypothesis to account for these parallels.[9] What Cuba's history shares with that of Jamaica, Taiwan, Sri Lanka, and Chile is the development or expansion of a similar system of economic organization at about the same time. All of these countries experienced substantial economic growth after World War I, when the expansion of world markets created a boom for the primary-goods export economies.[10] An important feature of these economies at the time was that the government sector made heavy expenditures to promote the growth of exports. As Birnberg and Resnick have noted,

The growth of trade experienced by these economies would hardly have been possible without expenditures on harbors, wharves, culverts, road systems, railroads, and other public works as well as investments in administrative infrastructure, in health facilities such as malaria and yellow fever control, in the establishment of order through an organized police and army, and in various productive agrarian activities such as irrigation, artesian wells, disease research for crops, and communication facilities.[11]

The significance of these developments as factors in reducing mortality is obvious, and it is very suggestive that these common elements may link the mortality decline observed in Cuba with similar changes in a number of other developing countries.

Further research on factors in the history of mortality in Cuba should attempt to define the influence of urbanization and of declining fertility. Some evidence discussed in this study suggests that both of these factors may have played important roles. The role of international efforts toward disease control (for example, the world-wide campaign against the spread of cholera during the first decades of this century) is also worth investigating. Although these internationally coordinated campaigns undoubtedly contributed to mortality decline from certain diseases in Cuba, as well as in other countries, it seems that their effect in Cuba would not have been so substantial had they not been complemented by strong efforts within the country.

Appendix 1: Evaluation of the Data

Nineteenth-Century Cuban Mortality Data

The total number of deaths by year has been recorded for the City of Havana almost uninterruptedly since 1801. I cannot establish the validity of such a series, although it probably conveys the more-conspicuous mortality fluctuations typical of nonmodern health conditions. In addition, statistics of deaths from typhoid and yellow fever in Havana date as far back as 1856, and of deaths from malaria, smallpox, tetanus, and tuberculosis as far back as the early 1870s.

If we contrast the data provided by different sources (apparently compiled independently), we can evaluate these statistics in a limited way. We can compare death-by-cause statistics that have survived for 1890 and 1891, with more limited compilations made available early in the 1900s.[1] Such comparison reveals that the total number of deaths and of deaths-by-cause in these sources are sufficiently similar for the nineteenth century so as not to invalidate their use in the analysis of gross tendencies of mortality change toward the end of the century.

Cuban Mortality Data from 1902 to 1953

Legal and Classificatory Aspects of Death Registration

In Cuba deaths were registered on a de facto basis. Since burial had to be within twenty-four hours, the death had to be reported immediately. By law, burial had to be in an officially approved public cemetery, after presentation of a license issued by the civil registration service. A prerequisite for the issuance of the burial permit (again, according to law) was the presentation of a medical certificate attesting that the death had occurred and stating the nature and cause of it.[2]

So-called fetal deaths and deaths occurring within twenty-four hours of birth were recorded as stillbirths. Under this system, a live birth was defined as the survival of a fetus having a "human" figure for at least twenty-four hours after complete separation from the mother.

Registration of vital events in Cuba was notoriously deficient, and, unfortunately, the legal requirements regarding death registration were constantly violated. Death registration was incomplete partly because of the separate registration of stillbirths and partly because the legal requirements for the medical certificates were difficult to meet.[3]

The existing death registration statistics collected from the 1902 to 1953 period have been tabulated by sex, race, age, and cause of death in general for each year for the country as a whole and for each province. They have been tabulated almost as frequently for the municipality of Havana (and for the City of Havana, exclusively, for 1901). In addition, the total numbers of deaths, tabulated by sex and race, are available for each municipality for each year. The age data were tabulated poorly in that the age groupings are not well suited to demographic analysis and are not standardized from period to period. The race dimension, following American usage as well as colonial practice, has been dichotomized into whites and nonwhites (colored), the latter group including not only blacks and mixed bloods, but also the population of Asian descent.

The death-by-cause statistics for the 1902-1953 period have been published in the official Cuban vital statistics journals according to the first six revisions of the International List of Causes of Death. Table 27 shows the years covered by each of the revisions, as well as the total number of causes of death under each revision as they appear in the Cuban publications. No statistics on death-by-cause were published for the years 1941 and 1942 for the country or for Havana, and after 1953 Cuban death-by-cause statistics were not published for a number of years. For the municipality of Havana in certain years, only the aggregated distribution of deaths-by-cause, combining the sex and race groupings, are shown in the official vital statistics journals from which I took my data.

The Completeness and Quality of Death Registration

We can assess the degree of completeness of death registration in Cuba only by indirect methods. Not only do the published statistics lack detailed tabulations for rigorous examination, but the unreliability of birth registration and the unknown quality of irregular population censuses complicate the problem. We cannot apply most conventional demographic techniques in these circumstances, without relying on weak assumptions. The uncertain recording of the large international migration experienced by the country during most of the twentieth century casts even more doubt on the reliability of formal techniques of demographic analysis. Nevertheless, researchers have attempted to use death-registration statistics, with substantially different results, because of some of the assumptions and methodology utilized.

On a priori grounds, we can assume that differential underregistration of deaths, both over time and across localities or regions, was the rule rather than the exception. In certain cases, regional differentials in the extent of registration can affect the analysis of mortality by causes. For example, if the reporting of deaths in areas where malaria was endemic was poorer than in areas where malaria was absent, the

Table 27
Revisions of International List of Causes of Death
Used by Cuban Statistical Service

Revision	Years Covered	Number of Causes of Death
First	1902-1909	179
Second	1910-1920	189
Third	1921-1929	205
Fourth	1930-1939	200
Fifth	1940-1949	200
Sixth	1950-1953	150

proportion of malaria-related deaths is understated.

Published Estimates of Completeness of Death Registration

Two sources provide estimates of the completeness of death registration in Cuba. Both have relied on the balancing equation, supplemented by theoretically or empirically derived estimates to fill gaps in the available information. The more ambitious effort has provided estimates of the completeness of the death register throughout the first half of the twentieth century.[4] The second study, which covers only the 1943-1953 census period, seems to provide better-grounded estimates.[5] Both sets, however, rest on debatable assumptions and tend to contradict one another.

O. Andrew Collver obtained his estimates in a study that derived a historical series of birth rates for the countries of Latin America. Collver's method was essentially an assessment of the consistency of birth and death registration, census and international migration data. In theory, if all three bodies of data were accurate, the recorded differences between natural increase and net migration would explain intercensal changes in the enumerated population. In practice, however, the quality of the data was rarely adequate to produce a close balance. This method assumed, however, that the major inconsistencies could be detected and corrected by substituting dependable estimates for the defective data segments. As Collver acknowledged, a major difficulty in the application of this technique was that compensating errors in the different sets of data were easily overlooked, since those errors could give results that appeared credible.

In spite of the biases that may have entered into Collver's estimates, it is worthwhile to comment on two other problems in his calculations. The first is the impact of immigration on the country's population, particularly during the first forty years that his estimates cover.[6] Although his estimates of net migration may represent the evidence provided by the movement-of-passenger statistics, historical sources indicate that that evidence underrepresents the true extent of net migration (the direction of the bias depending on the period in question). The statistics on movement of passengers may not reliably portray the actual flow and ebb of migration, because official statistics do not, of course, reflect entries of illegal migrants.[7]

The second problem in Collver's net-migration estimates arises from a statement he makes in a footnote: "The Cuban census of 1919 showed 18.5 percent foreign born, and by 1931 the percentage had increased to 23.0."[8] If Collver used percentages of foreign-born of that magnitude to obtain his estimates, the estimates are totally erroneous. Collver apparently made the mistake of confusing the foreign-born category with that of noncitizens. His estimate refers to the latter.[9]

Another significant technical problem in Collver's work relates to his assumptions concerning the levels of infant and child mortality (ages one to four). Although he was fully aware of the Cuban practice for registering stillbirths and was conscious of the deficiency of death registration as a result of the omission of large numbers of infant deaths, he assumed that the distribution of registered deaths by age was representative of the distribution of all deaths occurring in the country.[10] What is crucial is that he based that conclusion on an assumption derived from another assumption that was, in fact, the eventual conclusion. In my opinion, his assumptions lead to a severe underestimation of infant mortality and, consequently, to an unduly favorable estimate of the completeness of death registration and a probable understatement of fertility.

Table 28 shows Collver's estimates of the completeness of the Cuban death and birth registers in consecutive five-year periods. As we might have predicted, these estimates reflect a secular improvement that indicates nearly 90 percent completeness toward the end of the period.

The estimates by Fernando González Q. and Jorge Debasa, although similar in basic methodology to Collver's, relied on more sophisticated techniques and were based on more tenable assumptions. González and Debasa did not have to contend with uncertainties produced by international migration during the first four decades of the century, as Collver did, since, in the 1940-1950 decade, international migration was not as intense as in the earlier years. The González and Debasa estimates were obtained through the balancing equation, supplemented with mortality assumptions taken from published life tables from other Latin American countries, from model life-tables, and from estimates of survival probabilities derived from selected age-specific census survival-ratios computed from the Cuban censuses.

González and Debasa first proportionally distributed the registered deaths by age, according to the recorded experiences of Argentina, Chile, Mexico, and the United States, and allowed for two cohorts—those born during the intercensal period and those already alive by the time of the first census. They broke down the annual number of registered births by sex, according to a sex ratio at birth of 105 males per 100 females. Using the estimated number of registered deaths by age and sex (for each intercensal year) and the annual number of births by sex, they estimated the

Table 28
Collver's Estimates of Completeness of Death and Birth Registration, Cuba

Quinquennium	Ratio of Registered Events to Actual Number	
	Death Register	Birth Register
1900-1904	.633	.641
1905-1909	.631	.675
1910-1914	.656	.675
1915-1919	.663	.654
1920-1924	.729	.605
1925-1929	.787	.720
1930-1934	.837	.747
1935-1939	.860	.679
1940-1944	.887	—
1945-1949	.867	.757

Source: O. Andrew Collver, *Birth Rates in Latin America: New Estimates of Historical Trends and Fluctuations* (Berkeley: Institute of International Studies, University of California, 1965), pp. 38-39.

population as of 1 January 1953, with the starting base the enumerated population in 1943, adjusted to the beginning of the year (table 29). The resultant negative differences were what the authors had expected. Even greater differences would have resulted, however, had the compensatory effect of underregistration of both births and deaths not existed. The authors attributed the difference in sign for males and females over age ten to greater net immigration of females than of males during the census period.

Since the comparison of the two age distributions indicated that the five to nine age group had been accurately enumerated in the 1953 census, González and Debasa decided to estimate the actual number of births in 1948. They projected this age group backwards and utilized an adjusted set of survival values obtained through linear regressions that used as starting points the survival ratios found at ages thirty-five to thirty-nine with three different estimates of survival probabilities available for the intercensal period. The authors concluded that 90 percent of actual births were registered in 1948, assuming that the hypothesized mortality conditions were valid.

Finally, they used interpolations in United Nations model life-tables to evaluate the extent of death registration by determining central mortality rates that were assumed to reflect actual mortality conditions. They thus calculated an estimate of the numbers of deaths for the year 1948, and contrasted that number with the average number of registered deaths for 1947, 1948, and 1949 (see table 30).

Table 29
Estimated and Enumerated Population, 1 January 1953

Age	Enumerated Population	Estimated Population	Difference
Males			
0	70,596	79,896	− 9,300
1	70,496	80,834	−10,338
2	80,395	79,637	758
3	77,505	76,576	929
4	76,786	77,403	− 617
0-4	375,778	394,346	−18,568
5-9	363,271	362,351	920
0-9	739,049	756,697	−17,648
10 +	2,241,840	2,293,973	−52,133
Females			
0	67,934	76,614	− 8,680
1	67,052	77,440	−10,388
2	76,910	76,152	758
3	75,511	73,315	2,196
4	73,002	74,077	− 1,075
0-4	360,409	377,598	−17,189
5-9	348,694	347,469	1,225
0-9	709,067	−15,964	−15,964
10 +	2,129,724	2,107,822	21,902

Source: Fernando González Q. and Jorge Debasa, *Cuba: Evaluación y ajuste del censo de 1953 y las estadísticas de nacimientos y defunciones entre 1943 y 1958. Tabla de mortalidad por sexo, 1952-54*, Centro Latinoamericano de Demografía (CELADE), series C, no. 124 (Santiago: CELADE, 1970), p. 9.

As the table shows, the estimated underregistration of deaths was considerable. Infant and child deaths were more poorly recorded than adult deaths, and registration apparently was better for females than for males.

As tables 28 and 30 indicate, the two sets of estimates of completeness of death registration differ substantially for the years in which they are comparable. Collver's estimates have a wider range of variability than the more-limited estimates of González and Debasa, since the uncertainty in some variables is greater for the earlier part of the century.[11] The differences between the two series in the 1940-1950 decade are significant enough to investigate further. Since both sets of estimates begin with the same raw data, the alternative assumptions

Table 30
Comparative Death Statistics and Estimated Completeness
of Death Registration, 1948

Age	Estimated Number of Deaths	Average Number of Registered Deaths	Completeness of Death Registration (%)
Males			
0-4	14,694	5,101	34.71
5-14	1,704	712	41.78
15 +	23,749	16,443	69.24
Total	40,147	22,256	55.44
Females			
0-4	11,634	4,417	37.97
5-14	1,555	625	40.19
15 +	17,608	13,116	74.49
Total	30,797	18,158	58.96

Source: Fernando González Q. and Jorge Debasa, *Cuba: Evaluación y ajuste del censo de 1953 y las estadísticas de nacimientos y defunciones entre 1943 y 1958. Tabla de mortalidad por sexo, 1952-54*, Centro Latinoamericano de Demografía (CELADE), series C, no. 124 (Santiago: CELADE, 1970), p.14.

produced differences. We can assess the reasonableness of the two sets of estimates by comparing the adjusted crude rates derived from the estimated registration data with the unadjusted official rates. We can then compare the latter with unadjusted official rates of other countries in the region that have had fairly similar mortality experiences and whose statistics have been judged fairly reliable.[12] Tables 31 and 32 give estimated and official crude death rates for Cuba and for the comparison countries (by quinquennia and in single years).

As the tables show, during the years in which the sets of crude death rates are comparable, Collver's estimates are somewhat lower than the rates calculated by González and Debasa. The latter estimates appear to be in somewhat closer agreement with the rates presented for the comparison countries. Collver's estimates for the first twenty years of the century are substantially lower than the estimated crude death rates for British Guiana and Chile, but are very close to those given by G. W. Roberts for Jamaica.[13] By 1920 Collver's estimates begin to diverge from the values shown for the other countries. This period coincides with the era of heavy immigration into Cuba, and the estimates depend on what is regarded as the most-deficient of the modern Cuban censuses (1931). However, I am inclined to believe that the underestimated death rates and, thus, the underestimated completeness of

Table 31
Estimated and Official Crude Death Rates, 1900-1950

Quinquennium	Cuba (Collver)	Cuba (Official)	British Guiana	Chile	Costa Rica	Jamaica
1900-1904	23.7	13.7	—	31.4	—	22.7
1905-1909	23.3	14.5	—	31.6	—	25.0
1910-1914	21.4	13.6	27.0	29.8	—	22.8
1915-1919	22.2	14.8	33.1	31.0	—	26.9
1920-1924	19.3	14.4	26.8	30.1	—	23.5
1925-1929	15.2	12.1	24.6	25.8	24.7	19.6
1930-1934	13.3	10.9	22.5	24.7	23.2	18.3
1935-1939	12.7	10.4	20.9	24.0	19.8	16.1
1940-1944	10.9	9.9	18.4	19.9	18.5	—
1945-1949	8.7	8.3	14.5	16.4	13.8	—

Sources: *Cuba*—(Collver estimate) O. Andrew Collver, *Birth Rates in Latin America: New Estimates of Historical Trends and Fluctuations* (Berkeley: Institute of International Studies, University of California, 1965); (official rate) published figures on number of deaths and census data. *British Guiana*—Jay R. Mandle, "The Decline in Mortality in British Guiana, 1911-1960," *Demography* 7, no. 3 (August 1970):303. *Chile*—Markos Mamalakis, "Historical Statistics for Chile: 1840-1967," mimeographed, p. A-72, table IIA. *Costa Rica*—Earl E. Huyck, "Fecundidad y planificación familiar: El caso de Costa Rica," Quinto Seminario Nacional de Demografía (San José: Asociación Demográfica Costarricense, 1970), p. 476. *Jamaica*—G. W. Roberts, "A Note on Mortality in Jamaica," *Population Studies* 4, no. 1 (June 1950):69.

Notes: Official crude death rates computed from unadjusted registration and census data, per 1,000 population. The quinquennia for British Guiana, Chile, Costa Rica, and Jamaica are slightly different from those for Cuba in that they run one year later, that is, 1901-05, 1906-10, and so on. Dash signifies no data available.

Table 32
Estimated and Official Crude Death Rates, 1943-1953

Year	Crude Death Rate				
	Cuba (González and Debasa)	(Official)	British Guiana	Chile	Costa Rica
1943	17.7	10.4	n.a.	19.9	18.4
1944	16.9	9.9	21.9	19.5	17.3
1945	17.8	10.4	17.8	20.0	16.0
1946	13.6	8.0	15.7	17.0	14.4
1947	13.3	7.8	14.7	16.1	15.4
1948	12.9	7.6	14.3	16.7	13.5
1949	12.8	7.5	13.2	17.3	13.1
1950	12.1	7.1	14.6	15.0	12.5
1951	12.4	7.3	13.3	15.0	11.9
1952	11.0	6.5	n.a.	13.0	11.8
1953	10.8	6.4	12.5	12.4	11.0

Sources: *Cuba*—Fernando González Q. and Jorge Debasa, *Cuba: Evaluación y ajuste del censo de 1953 y las estadísticas de nacimientos y defunciones entre 1943 y 1958. Tabla de mortalidad por sexo, 1952-54*, Centro Latinoamericano de Demografía (CELADE), series C, no. 124 (Santiago: CELADE, 1970), p. 29.
Other countries—same as for table 31.
Note: Official crude death rate computed from unadjusted registration and census data, per 1,000 population.

the death register, are mainly the result of the unrealistically low infant- and child-mortality assumptions that Collver made. It must be noted, however, that differences in age structures and levels of fertility may influence a comparison of the levels of the death rates across countries. For example, if Cuba's birth rate were lower than Jamaica's, different age structures would emerge that would produce different crude death rates even under similar age-specific mortality.

Based on the above comparison and on my assessment of the estimating procedures used in the two studies, I conclude that the estimates of completeness made by González and Debasa appear to be closer to reality than those by Collver. Furthermore, I conclude that early in the century, death registration was not higher than 30 to 40 percent complete nationwide and gradually improved to the levels estimated by González and Debasa for the 1940s. The overall range of completeness of death registration for the first half of the century is between 30 and 60 percent, but probably does not exceed 50 percent.

Death Statistics for Havana: Special Considerations

A series of death-by-cause statistics parallel to the one for the republic has been published each year for the municipality of Havana from 1901 to 1953 (such statistics were first published for Cuba in 1902). Since deaths were registered in Cuba on a de facto basis, many of the deaths registered in Havana were probably of nonresidents. Certainly many residents of areas immediately surrounding Havana, as well as some from other parts of the country, sought the superior and highly concentrated medical facilities the city had to offer. We cannot estimate the extent to which the registration of nonresident deaths affects the recorded mortality rates, since tabulations of deaths by place of residence do not exist.

Death registration in the capital was virtually complete, if Cuban experience was similar to that of many other countries. Laws and regulations are more likely to be adhered to in a country's capital, and the majority of deaths take place in or are processed through institutions (hospitals, cemeteries) that properly register all deaths and their causes.

Another difficulty in the use of the Havana death statistics is that the municipality of Havana did not contain the whole metropolitan area from which the centrally located medical facilities drew many patients. According to the 1953 census, metropolitan Havana included the urbanized sections of the municipalities of Bauta, Guanabacoa, Havana proper, Marianao, Regla, Santa María del Rosario, and Santiago de las Vegas.[14] The death-by-cause statistics are provided by municipality for most years, but are never broken down by urban and rural sectors. We can get some indication of the effect of registration of deaths from the whole metropolitan region of Havana on the overall level of death registration in the municipality if we compare the crude death rates for the municipality with the rates that result from combining the data for all the municipalities within the metropolitan area. Table 33 presents the absolute figures for registered deaths and enumerated population in each census year and the resulting crude death rates for each area.

As table 33 indicates, the crude death rates for the two areas have almost identical values for each of the census years except 1953. This closeness appears to mean that the counterbalancing forces resulting from registering deaths by place of occurrence cancel each other out. However, such an assumption is unwarranted as regards the death-by-cause rates, in view of comments made earlier. In fact, we can conclude nothing with any certainty with respect to the effects of the counterbalancing forces on the distribution of deaths-by-cause.

We can make another comparison if we observe what percentage of all deaths registered in the country was recorded in the municipality of Havana or in the metropolitan area (see table 34). Not surprisingly, the percentages of deaths registered in the two areas exceed the corresponding percentages of the total population found in the areas because of the overregistration resulting from the deaths of nonresidents there and because of the superior registration in the Havana area and the very high levels of underregistration estimated for the rest of the country. Differences in age structure between the Havana region and the rest of the country and differences in levels of actual age-specific death rates for the two areas may affect these comparisons.

Table 33

Population, Number of Registered Deaths, and Crude Death Rates

Census Year	Municipality of Havana			Metropolitan Havana		
	Number Registered Deaths	Population	Crude Death Rate	Number Registered Deaths	Population	Crude Death Rate
1907	6,708	302,526	22.2	8,164	376,053	21.7
1919	7,629	363,506	21.0	9,926	476,369	20.8
1931	7,988	542,522	14.7	10,836	733,738	14.8
1943	9,694	676,376	14.3	13,522	956,321	14.1
1953	8,425	787,765	10.7	11,227	1,240,369	9.9

Source: Cuban censuses and vital statistics.

Table 34

Percentage of National Total of Registered Deaths and of Total Population

Census Year	Municipality of Havana		Metropolitan Havana	
	Deaths	Population	Deaths	Population
1907	19.7	14.8	24.0	18.4
1919	18.5	12.6	24.1	16.5
1931	19.8	13.7	25.8	18.5
1943	19.4	14.2	27.1	20.0
1953	22.7	13.5	30.2	21.3

Source: Cuban censuses and vital statistics.

We can draw few conclusions with respect to the correspondence between the base population and the registered deaths because of the way in which deaths were recorded. However, because we assume fuller death registration in the municipality and very low percentages of ill-defined causes of death in the city, we can hypothesize that the mortality data for Havana represent a good standard against which to judge the reasonableness of death registration in the rest of the country. Unfortunately, we do not know the effect that reporting of deaths by place of occurrence may have had on the patterns of death-by-cause and on the overall distribution of the patterns.

Evaluation of Post-1953 Cuban Mortality Data

After 1953 and up to the early sixties, hardly any demographic statistics were made available for Cuba.[15] In the late 1960s, demographic statistics were published, and in the 1970s, Cuban mortality statistics were regularly issued. The assessment made by the Comité Estatal de Estadísticas of mortality conditions in the country in 1970 includes a discussion of the national death-registration system and some of its shortcomings.[16] To my knowledge, no detailed evaluation of the death statistics for recent years has been made public, although the comité's report indicates that some yet-to-be-published studies have been conducted, and there are strong indications that mortality data have achieved a high degree of reliability. As Vincente Navarro assesses the improvements,

It is to the credit of the new Cuban government that, especially since 1965, high priority has been placed on establishing a reliable system of data gathering within the health sector in order to cover the whole population. The result of this policy can be seen in the area of death registration, where, for example, only 53 percent of all deaths in Cuba were reported in 1956 (in rural areas the figure was even lower, where only 30 percent were reported); but by 1969, 98 percent of all deaths in the country were reported and documented with medical certificates.[17]

My evidence supports this and similar assessments. In general, the data available since the late 1960s appears to be of exceptional quality, particularly for a developing country.

Evaluation of the Census Data

No formal effort has been made in this study to evaluate the Cuban censuses. In general, they appear to be of acceptable quality, with the exception of heavy underenumeration of children under two years of age (as noted by Collver). The Centro Latinoamericano de Demografía has evaluated some aspects of the censuses of 1919, 1931, 1943, and 1953,[18] and, according to the results of a postenumeration survey conducted after the 1970 census, that census was exceptionally reliable.[19] The Cuban censuses of 1899 and 1907, although superficially analyzed in subsequent census volumes, have not been studied in great detail.

Conclusions regarding the Quality of Cuban Mortality Data

We can reach a number of conclusions based on the preceding evaluation of available Cuban demographic statistics. First, the nature and quality of the information varies considerably from period to period. Second, even in those periods for which the data are most deficient, they are sufficiently revealing to give some indication of what the mortality trends were. Third, the data for the City of Havana appear to be reliable enough to allow us to study the determinants of the mortality transition there with some rigor. We can also use the information from Havana to make inferences regarding the course of events in the rest of the country, although we do not presume that exactly similar mortality conditions prevailed in Havana and in Cuba as a whole. Judicious assessments coupled with the ever-present recognition of data limitations can help us reach an understanding of the conditions that led to the decline of mortality in Cuba.

Appendix 2: Adjustments in the Data

The population estimates described in this appendix are not intended for use in very refined demographic evaluation, but rather as a basis for the calculation of the mortality rates used in this study. Errors in these estimates are not likely to alter the picture of mortality trends significantly, even if, at some points, the picture of changing population structure may be distorted.

Intercensal Population Estimates for the City of Havana

I used linear interpolation between successive censuses to obtain the population estimates needed to derive the series of crude death rates for Havana. Although this method tends to overestimate the population for the years closer to the first census and to underestimate it for the years closer to the second, I believe that a more elaborate method would not have resulted in more precision, because of Cuba's experience of cyclical international migrations during the 1880-1953 period. These migrations affected the size of the population significantly over short periods of time, especially in local areas within the country.

The benchmarks I used to estimate the population of Havana before the census of 1899 were the figures obtained in the Spanish censuses of 1877 and 1887, censuses that provide data on the city's population. I obtained the intercensal estimates of Havana's population during the twentieth century by using data on the municipality rather than on the city, because the censuses of 1931 and 1953 give data only for the municipality, and because the numbers of deaths given for most of the census years refer to the municipality.

Population Figures for Havana Used To Derive Age-Specific Mortality Measurements

The censuses of 1899, 1907, 1919, and 1931 give separate total population figures for the city and for the municipality, but provide sex and age breakdown for the city only. Hence, I used city figures to compute age-specific mortality measures. The census of 1943, on the other hand, gives the sex and age distributions for both the city and the municipality. I used the 1943 municipality data, since they are more easily adjustable to obtain a finer age distribution. The 1953 census gives the sex and age data only for the municipality.

Although I expected minor biases from the switch between municipality and city data, I saw no other option. Besides, the biases should not be very large, since, by the time of the two most-recent censuses, the city extended practically over the entire municipality. Table 35 shows the enumerated population of the city and of the municipality at each census date, as well as the population of the city as a percentage of the population of the municipality.

Table 35
City of Havana Population as Percentage
of Municipality of Havana Population

Census Year	Population of City	Population of Municipality	City Population as % of Municipality Population
1899	235,981	253,418	93.0
1907	297,159	302,526	98.2
1919	363,506[a]	363,506	100.0
1931	520,504	542,522	95.9
1943	659,883	676,376	97.6
1953	—[b]	787,765	100.0

[a] I presume that in 1919 the census authorities assumed that the population of the City of Havana corresponded to that of the municipality.

[b] No data available for the city. I have assumed that in 1953 the population of the city was the same as the population of the municipality.

Adjustments to the Census Data for the City of Havana

1901 Census

I estimated the total population of the city in 1901 (no census was taken in that year) by using linear interpolation of the enumerated population in 1899 and the population adjusted for the underenumeration of children under age one in 1907. A more-sophisticated estimating technique would not have increased the precision of my estimate, since voluminous, unrecorded population changes probably took place in the city during the years immediately following the cessation of hostilities. I distributed the total estimated population according to the proportionate age and sex structure recorded in the 1899 census. Instead of using the population under one year of age enumerated in the 1899 census, I substituted the average number of registered births recorded in the years 1900, 1901, and 1902 (not available by sex) and distributed those averages according to a sex ratio of 102 males per 100 females. I did this because there is evidence of a large increase in fertility following the 1895-1898 war and because it seems that during these years birth registration was virtually complete in Havana. The sex ratio of 102 was used because this was the sex ratio recorded in 1907, a census year in which the more balanced and complete registration of births by sex was recorded. I followed this procedure because it is obvious that the Cuban censuses suffer from heavy underenumeration of young children. This substitution increased the size of the population under one year and, hence, the size of the total population. The substitution of births for the estimated population under one year of age was justified by my assumption that the reduction in the population size under one year of age due to mortality was equivalent to the reduction resulting from underregistration of births. I believe that this statistical manipulation minimizes, for the estimated infant-mortality rates, the biases that would occur because of severe underenumeration of children under one year of age.

I made no attempt to correct the age group one to four, although it is almost certain that the population estimate in that age range understates the actual numbers. Since the one to four age group in 1901 included cohorts born during and after the war period, and since no firm guidelines existed for adjusting this age group, I decided to leave it as originally estimated. A bias results, but of an unknown magnitude.

1907 Census

I accepted the enumerated population of the city as given (the unknown ages were proportionally distributed across all ages), with the exception of the data for children under one year of age. For that age group, I substituted the number of births recorded for each sex in 1907. This correction procedure may tend to produce lower estimates of infant mortality than should, in reality, be expected. In this case, I used birth-registration statistics for only one year, rather than the average number of births for the years surrounding the census year. Because it was common in Cuba for births to be registered late (often the government granted grace periods during which births previously unregistered were recorded), the estimate might have been affected by an erratic swing in the annual number of registered births (they were published by year of registration rather than by year of occurrence). I attempted no adjustments in the data for ages one to four, although it is likely that the population at those ages was also underenumerated.

1919 Census

With the exception of correcting for underenumeration of children under one year of age, I accepted the age-sex structure for this year as shown in the 1919 census. For children under one year of age, I based my estimate on the numer of registered births in 1919. I inflated the number of registered female births to obtain a sex ratio of 102, equal to that of 1907 (differential underregistration of female births was suggested by a sex ratio of registered births of 111). Again this adjustment procedure seems to overcompensate for the underenumeration of children under the age of one. Although there is some evidence of underenumeration at ages one through four, I made no attempt to correct for it. The population of unknown ages was proportionally distributed across all ages.

1931 Census

I again substituted the number of registered births during the census year for the number of children under one year of age. I inflated the number of registered female births to match the sex ratio in 1907 (the sex ratio in 1931 was 112). The same bias produced in the figures for 1907 and 1919 should be expected from this procedure. No population of unknown ages was recorded in this census.

I had to manipulate the raw data from this census in order to derive the five-year age groups needed for the computation of life tables. The data for the age groups one to four and five to nine were directly available. I obtained the estimated populations at ages ten to fourteen and fifteen to nineteen by combining the age group ten to thirteen with an estimate of the population at age fourteen (calculated by subtracting one-fourth of the age group ten to thirteen from the age group fourteen to nineteen). I based this estimating procedure on the assumption of very low mortality at those ages and no migration.

Above age twenty, only ten-year age groupings were given in the 1931 census. I therefore estimated five-year age groups by distributing the population in each ten-year age group according to the average distribution between the component five-year age groups in the 1919 and 1953 censuses. This procedure should not result in large distortions.

1943 Census

I had to make the most considerable and questionable adjustments to the age data provided by this census. For some reason (probably to save space, since for the first time in the Cuban censuses, the age distribution for each municipality was shown), the population by sex was distributed in very unconventional and analytically unwieldy age groups (under five, five to thirteen, fourteen to nineteen, twenty to forty-nine, and fifty and over). In order to derive a convenient five-year age distribution, I followed a number of steps. I distributed the population under five years of age in two age groups (under one and one to four) by linearly interpolating their proportionate shares in the total under age five between the adjusted population for the City of Havana in 1931 and that of the municipality of Havana in 1953. I made no attempt to correct for possible bias in the estimate of population under one year of age after this manipulation. I then converted the age groups five to thirteen and fourteen to nineteen into age groups of five to fourteen and fifteen to nineteen by adding or substracting the population of fourteen years of age (obtained from an enumerated population of school age by single years given for the municipality). I divided the five to fourteen age group into two quinquennial segments by a procedure similar to the one used with the population under five years of age.

I first divided the population twenty to forty-nine into three ten-year age segments by linearly interpolating their proportionate shares in the thirty-year total between the 1931 census (where only ten-year groupings are given) and the 1953 census. Finally, I divided the estimated ten-year age groups into five-year groups, according to the distribution of the 1953 quinquennial groupings. I used a similar procedure for the population above age fifty.

Unfortunately, a large portion of my analysis depends on the estimated age structure of Havana's population of each sex in 1943. I used these age structures to derive the life tables for that year and also as the standards against which to calculate cause-specific-age and age-sex-standardized death rates. The selection of these estimated age structures as standards was necessary, since the statistics of death by cause for 1943 (or for any other year in the 1940 decade) were not published by age. By using the estimated 1943 age structures as the standards, I was able to obtain a directly standardized series of age-sex-specific death rates that included the year 1943, since with all other years standardized to 1943, I could use the 1943 death data without an age breakdown. Despite the uncertainties, the benefits outweigh the disadvantages because otherwise the series of age and age-sex-standardized cause-specific death rates would have had a twenty-two-year gap (1931-1953) during a period in which drastic mortality changes took place.

1953 Census

Except for prorating the population of ages unknown, I made no adjustments to the data for this census.

Adjustments to the Census Data for Cuba

1907 Census

I used the average of the estimated rate of growth for the native white-female population in ages ten to forty-nine and fifteen to forty-nine between the census years of 1899 and 1907 to project that population forward to 1909. This manipulation allowed me to derive life expectancy estimates for the periods 1899 to 1909, and 1909 to 1919, since the model life-table estimating techniques that I applied to the data given by the censuses of 1899, 1907, and 1919, required ten-year intervals between the dates of population counts.

Adjustments to the Death Statistics for Havana

In order to compute my life tables for the City of Havana, I made some adjustments to the published death statistics at particular dates, mainly because they were not available in sufficient detail for age. In each censal period separate statistics are given for the age groups under one and one to four. However, I could obtain data in five-year age groups only for dates around the censuses of 1919 and 1931. For other census years, as table 36 shows, data were provided only in broad age groups, varying from period to period.

Table 36
Age Distributions for Death Statistics, Municipality of Havana

1901	1907	1919	1953
0-1	0-1	0-1	0-1
1-4	1-4	1-4	1-4
5-9	5-14	5-9	5-9
10-19	15-29	10-14	15-24
20-39	30-44	15-19	25-44
40-59	45-59	20-39	45-64
60-69	60-74	40-59	65-74
70+	70+	60+	75+

Notes: For 1919 and 1931, the death statistics by sex and race, but not by cause, are given for Havana in five-year age groups. Deaths by sex, race, and cause are given for those two years as shown in the column for 1919.

Death statistics for 1940, 1944, and 1945 are available by sex and race, but not by cause, in the same age distribution as that for 1919.

In order to derive five-year age groups for the needed years, I assumed that the deaths in any given period were internally distributed within the given broad age-range according to the average of the distributions of the deaths around 1919 and 1931. For example, I broke down the numbers of deaths in 1953 at ages twenty-five to forty-four according to the average proportional distribution of the deaths in ages twenty-five to twenty-nine, thirty to thirty-four, thirty-five to thirty-nine, and forty to forty-four within the age group twenty-five to forty-four in 1918-1920 and 1930-1932.

This procedure may somewhat distort the distribution of deaths by age for those periods in which the actual distributions were not shown, particularly if mortality conditions had changed radically or if the age distributions of the population had become significantly different from those observed in 1919 and 1931. These are credible possibilities, since we are dealing with an urban population subjected to cyclical currents of international migration and also experiencing heavy in-migration. We may expect additional changes in the age distribution from the declines in both secular fertility and mortality that Cuba has experienced.

Table 37 presents the percentage distributions of the enumerated or estimated male population of Havana in five-year age groups above age five. (Changes below age five are not relevant, since, for every period, deaths are listed separately for the age groups under that age.) Although the changes in the age structure were substantial, they do not appear to have been great enough to cause gross errors in the

Table 37
Percentage Distribution of Male Population Over Age Five,
Municipality of Havana

Age Group	Census Year					
	1899	1907	1919	1931	1943	1953
5-9	10.5	8.6	10.5	9.5	8.6	8.4
10-14	10.1	8.2	9.8	9.0	8.4	8.4
15-19	11.0	13.0	12.0	9.2	8.2	7.9
20-24	13.2	15.1	11.2	12.8	11.5	10.2
25-29	13.1	13.2	12.1	12.8	11.2	9.9
30-34	10.9	10.8	11.1	10.6	9.8	9.3
35-39	8.6	8.8	9.2	9.0	8.8	8.2
40-44	6.9	7.0	7.0	7.7	8.1	8.4
45-49	4.7	5.0	5.5	6.5	7.7	8.0
50-54	4.2	3.8	4.4	4.8	6.0	6.8
55-59	2.6	2.3	2.7	3.0	3.9	4.3
60-64	2.1	2.0	2.0	2.3	3.3	4.3
65-69	1.0	0.9	1.0	1.3	2.1	2.7
70-74	0.6	0.7	0.7	0.6	1.2	1.7
75-79	0.2	0.3	0.4	0.5	0.7	0.9
80-84	0.1	0.2	0.2	0.2	0.3	0.4
85+	0.1	0.1	0.1	0.1	0.2	0.2
Total	100.0	100.0	100.0	100.0	100.0	100.0

estimates of age distribution of deaths. Since I distributed the numbers of deaths in the unknown five-year groups according to the known proportions within broad age ranges, we should not expect very large errors.

The distribution of deaths for 1943 also had to be estimated, since deaths by age were not published for that year (only the total number of deaths and the distributions by cause, sex, and race). Data on the number of deaths distributed by age, however, were available for 1940, 1944, and 1945, and thus the average of the numbers of deaths by age for those years was used to approximate that of 1943. I used the distribution of deaths by cause and by sex given for 1943 to estimate cause-specific rates.

Appendix 3: Sources and Evaluation of the Life Tables for Havana and Cuba

I computed life tables by sex and for both sexes combined for Havana at six dates. I derived the earliest one (1901) by projecting the enumerated 1899 population of the city to 1901, and by relating the estimated population to the death statistics (first published in that year in sufficient detail). I calculated the remaining life tables by relating population counts of the years 1907, 1919, 1931, 1943, and 1953 to the death statistics for those years or surrounding years. I made some adjustments to the data in order to compute these life tables, but I did not smooth them. Thus they show certain irregularities associated with biases in the raw data (See Appendix 2 for details of the adjustments). I obtained all of the Havana life tables by similar methods.[1]

The most serious shortcoming of the life tables for Havana is that they have been estimated using deaths registered on a de facto basis and the enumerated population of the city, which method results in a tendency to overestimate the actual mortality levels. The adjustments made to the population and death data may have introduced additional minor biases. However, it is unlikely that these biases distort the actual secular trend of mortality. The most significant bias appears to have resulted from adjusting the Havana population under one year of age for the years 1907, 1919, and 1931 (see Appendix 2). Because of these adjustments, the resultant infant mortality rates for these years are unduly low.

However, the basic outline of the mortality trends remains unchanged, as we can ascertain by inspecting a series (not shown) computed with the unadjusted data. The Havana infant-mortality estimates overall appear too low (in relation to comparable values in model life-tables). Heavy registration of de facto deaths in the city probably compensates to an unknown extent for the low infant mortality estimates, as far as the life expectancy estimates are concerned. The same biases apply particularly to the estimates of cause-specific mortality that specifically affect young children. Again, although biases are present, they do not distort the trends nor do they distort the interpretations of the causative factors.

The series of life tables for Cuba was composed of published life tables and estimated life tables. I estimated the two earliest life tables (1899 to 1909, and 1909 to 1919) by means of life-table models as explained below. Students from the Centro Latinoamericano de Demografía have derived life tables for the years 1919-1931, 1931-1943, and 1952-1954.[2] Official life tables are available for 1970.[3] Other life tables for intermediate dates have been computed on the basis of the ones just described (see table 3).

The 1919-1931 and 1931-1943 life tables were calculated by estimating census survival ratios after attempting to remove the effects of international migration from the age distributions. The life tables for 1953 (1952-1954) were obtained by the more conventional method of relating recorded deaths to population after adjusting the enumerated age structure and correcting for severe underregistration of deaths.

I computed the life tables for 1899-1909 and 1909-1919 by first projecting the 1907 enumerated native white-female population to 1909, in order to have the two ten-year intervals required to apply the model life-tables survival rates (which are given in five-year age groupings).[4] Because international migration was a very important factor in the dynamics of the Cuban population early in the century, I derived the estimates by using the data for natives (which may be considered a more-or-less closed segment). I had to exclude the nonwhites at the outset, since the Cuban censuses do not provide a distinction based on nativity for this subgroup, although nonwhites constituted a fairly sizable portion of the population at the time. Inspection by sex of the age structures revealed that the statistics for native white-males were distorted by peculiar biases in enumeration or by the inclusion of either foreign-born whites or nonwhites in the native white category, or by the inclusion of both. Therefore, I used the native white-female age structures exclusively to derive the estimates, and I assumed that the sex mortality differentials implied by the model life-tables applied to Cuba. I obtained the life table for both sexes by averaging the corresponding values for each sex, without attempting any adjustments for proportional representation. I decided on theoretical, as well as empirical, grounds to rely on the South model life-tables of Ansley Coale's and Paul Demeny's regional models.[5] Jeremiah Sullivan demonstrated that the South family is likely to give sounder estimates than those obtained using Coale's and Demeny's West regional family for developing countries, in which infant mortality is substantially higher than in the western European countries from whose experience the West model life-tables are derived.[6] Both regional sets of model life-tables were tested, and the South family provided estimates of life expectancy at birth about 8 percent lower than did the West family. The values derived with the South model show a pattern consistent with the later life-tables. I have accepted these two life tables (1899-1909 and 1909-1919) as indicative of the mortality levels within a broad range.

The q_x values for the Cuba life tables (see Appendix 5) suggest that some biases or defects may have entered into the estimation of one or more of the life-table sets. The reliability of the life tables for Cuba is explored below.

The close correspondence of the q_x values for 1905 (1899-1909) and 1915 (1909-1919) is not surprising, since I derived them by interpolating closely spaced values of the Coale and Demeny model life-tables. Critical is whether these two intercensal estimates approximate the real mortality conditions prevalent at the time, and, if not, why not? Since I derived these estimates from the comparison of successive age-structures, I had first to determine the extent to which the enumerated (or estimated) age structures conformed to the actual population of native white-females. The most likely source of bias was underenumeration in the censuses. If we hypothesize serious underenumeration in only one of the three censuses in question, the respective q_x values should deviate significantly if the mortality conditions remained unchanged (the data for Havana suggest that no great changes in mortality occurred during the first two decades of the century). If we assume that the defective census was the middle one, the results would indicate different mortality conditions, since we would have underestimated mortality in the first intercensal period, but overestimated it in the second. The following illustrates how a deficient census would have affected the mortality estimates.

First census	First estimate	Second census	Second estimate	Third census
accurate	within range	accurate	overestimate	deficient
accurate	overestimate	deficient	underestimate	accurate
deficient	underestimate	accurate	within range	accurate

Undercounts in all three censuses, unless differentially large, should not have affected the estimates significantly, since the bias in one census would cancel the biases in the others. Deficiencies in two censuses, but not in the third, could hardly have produced q_x values lying within so close a range. Under fairly stable mortality conditions, different patterns would have emerged, since, regardless of the position of the accurate census, over- or underestimates of mortality would have resulted.

Another issue in the reliability of Cuban life tables is whether the mortality experience of the native white-female population truly represents the mortality conditions for the total population. On theoretical grounds we can argue that an estimate based on this segment of the total population would understate the actual mortality level. In the first place, I believe that some of the immigrants arriving at the time in Cuba had a higher mortality rate than the natives'. If this is true, then the male-female relationship embodied in the model life-tables would tend to understate the true mortality levels, since most of the immigrants were males.

The nonnative whites may not have differed substantially from the native whites, partly because both groups shared the same basic living conditions and also because they originated primarily in countries with higher life expectancies than Cuba's (mainly Spain). But since the nonwhites accounted for about 30 percent of the total population and since they presumably experienced heavier mortality, it follows that the estimates may present an overly optimistic picture.

Except for the reservations regarding the representativeness of the native white population, we can confidently dismiss all the other considerations. For one thing, the Cuban censuses are fairly dependable, with the exception of that of 1931 (not included in the estimates) and except for the heavy underenumeration in all censuses of children under age two. Moreover, my estimating method, although only approximate, minimizes the impact of any one segment of the age structure on the selection of the most likely mortality level by relying on the use of the cumulative age distribution (ogive). Whereas these considerations may not conclusively show the 1905 and 1915 estimates to be acceptable, certain peculiarities observed in the 1925 (1919-1931) and 1937 (1931-1943) life tables suggest that more serious reservations exist about the validity of the later estimates than about the earlier ones.

One important characteristic of the 1925 and 1937 life tables is that the q_x values at ages zero and five are substantially lower than the corresponding values in the 1905 and 1915 life tables. Such a relationship is consistent with a secular trend of mortality decline. It is important to recall that empirical evidence has demonstrated a strong relationship between the different age segments of a mortality schedule. Coale's and Demeny's widely used model life-tables, which define four such possible relationships in the regional tables, embody this principle. Whatever the relationship, researchers have found that, generally, the higher the mortality rates in infancy and childhood, the higher they are in the rest of the age schedule, and vice versa.

In the life tables for 1925 and 1937 calculated at the Centro Latinoamericano de Demografía (CELADE), this basic principle is patently violated by the q_x schedule. Figure 19 compares the q_x values of the 1925 CELADE life table with the likely ranges of q_x schedules as defined by the four Coale and Demeny regional tables at a similar level of life expectancy (all of the curves refer to females). We can see that the 1925 q_x curve conforms to the models' pattern at the earliest ages, but that it differs radically at all other ages. It exceeds the overall q_x levels at the middle ages and lies at lower levels toward the older ages.

In order to identify the source of error, I reviewed the methodology followed in the calculation of the 1925 and 1937 life tables. The basic procedure derived census survival-ratios after removing the effects of international migration, and thus estimated the ratios for a supposedly closed population. Since the foreign born constituted a sizable percentage of the total population in 1919, 1931, and 1943 (11.7, 11.0, and 5.2 percent, respectively), the error probably occurred in the migration component.

In fact, it is likely that several of the assumptions tended to exaggerate mortality in the middle range of the age schedule and minimize it toward the older ages. Since the author of the CELADE study did not have the age distribution of all the foreign born, he assumed that their age distribution in both the 1919 and 1931 censuses was similar to that of the foreign-born population enumerated in the 1947 Argentinean census.[7] He reasoned that Argentina's immigration history was very similar to Cuba's. However, the assumption did not take into account the timing of the migrations. By 1947 international migration had already passed its peak in Argentina. Cuba experienced its highest levels of immigration in 1919 and somewhat again in 1931. In both Cuba and Argentina, the heaviest immigration occurred early in the century. By 1947 many of the foreign born in Argentina were no longer in the prime migratory ages (fifteen to forty-four). However, in Cuba in 1919, but less so by 1931, the foreign born, who had reached Cuban shores in large numbers during the economic expansion of the first three decades of the century, tended to be younger.

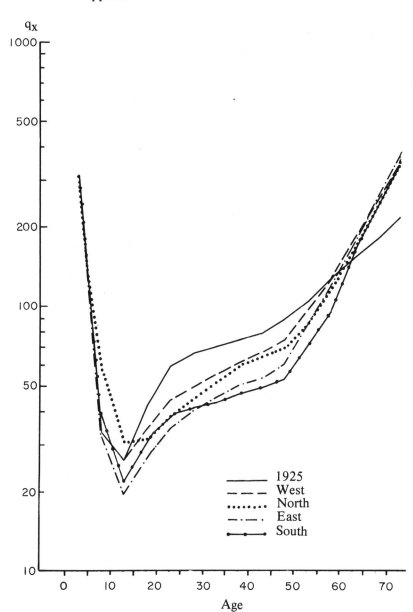

Figure 19. Female q_x Curves from 1925 Cuban Life Table and from Regional Model Life-Tables (Life Expectancy at Birth, 40 Years)

Table 38 shows that nearly 72 percent of the foreign-born white males enumerated in the 1919 census of Cuba were in the fifteen to forty-four age group. By contrast, only 37 percent of the foreign-born males were in that age range by 1947 in Argentina. It is also probable that in Cuba in 1919, the concentration of the foreign born in the fifteen to forty-four age range was even more intense, since the nonwhite immigrants had been permitted to enter the country only during the years immediately preceding the census.

Table 38

Age Distribution of Foreign-Born White Males

(Percentages)

Age Group	Cuba (1919)	Argentina (1947)
0-14	4.9	1.5
15-44	71.6	37.2
45+	23.4	61.3

Sources: *Cuba—1919 Census of Population*, table 8, p. 418. *Argentina*—Rodolfo Mezquita, *Cuba: Estimación de la mortalidad por sexo. Tabla de vida para los períodos 1919-31 y 1931-43*, series C, no. 121 (Santiago, Chile: Centro Latinoamericano de Demografía, June 1970), table 3, p. 22.

The bias introduced by this assumption concerning the foreign-born age distribution is evident, since this erroneous assumption was used to estimate the numbers of migrants who had entered or departed the country during the two intercensal periods. The CELADE study's author aged foreign born enumerated in each census according to a mortality schedule derived by weighting proportionally the known or assumed mortality conditions of the areas from which the migrants had originated. The difference between the survivors of the original foreign-born cohorts (for 1919-31, the 1919 survivors, and for 1931-43, the 1931 survivors) and the number of enumerated foreign born in the second census (the 1931 or the 1943 census) represented the effects of net international migration. For the first intercensal period, the difference was positive, indicating net immigration; for the second, negative, indicating net emigration. Depending on the outcome of this procedure, the author subtracted the estimated number of migrants from or added it to the number of foreign born enumerated in the second census, according to the model tables of migration-age structure prepared by the United Nations.[8] In these migration models, the migrants are heavily concentrated in the middle range of the age structure.

The effects of the statistical manipulations just described tend, first, to overestimate the total number of immigrants, since the foreign born are heavily weighted toward the older ages, where the force of mortality is strongest. The result is the disproportionate removal across the age range of many surviving nonnatives and, possibly, of some of the surviving natives as well. Second, the effects distort further because, in removing the estimated number of immigrants, the model migration-age structure favoring the younger ages is used. The result is that the calculated number of survivors is understated up to about age sixty and overstated above that age. Therefore, when we calculate census survival rates from the supposedly closed age-structures, the rates exaggerate the mortality levels up to about age sixty, but underestimate them above that age. These are precisely the deviations that the 1925 life tables show. Since the overestimated q_x values proportionally surpass the underestimated q_x values at the older ages, the life expectancies at most ages given by this set of life tables are too low (assuming no other significant problems).

Although similar defects characterize the 1937 life tables, the changing circumstances by that period make the evaluation of these life tables extremely difficult. In the first place, the proportion of foreign born in the 1943 census was considerably lower than in the earlier censuses. In the second place, a sizable emigration occurred between 1931 and 1943. If the effects of emigration ran in the opposite direction to those produced by immigration, we would expect the exact reversal of the pattern observed in the 1925 life tables. However, this does not occur. In figure 20 the female q_x curve for 1937 is plotted against the range of q_x curves defined by the four families of regional model life-tables at approximate levels of life expectancy at birth, and the same bias appears again. Still, the deviations for this life table are reduced, in comparison to deviations in earlier life tables. It is striking to see that the $_5q_0$ value given by this life table is lower than that given by even the West model life-table at a similar level of life expectancy at birth, and it is about 20 percent lower than that of the 1925 life table.

By 1931 the average age of nonnative population was probably higher than the average in 1919, since migrants had stopped coming some years earlier. This factor alone tends to minimize the errors. Finally, if we postulate that the most recent migrants were the most likely to leave Cuba under adverse economic conditions, it follows that the younger migrants must have been disproportionly represented among those who left, even more than assumed by the model emigration-age structure. This would explain the apparent overestimate of mortality at the younger ages for the second interval.

We can accept the life tables for Cuba in 1953 as fairly reliable (I discuss the methodology used in estimating these life tables in Appendix 1). We can also accept the reliability of the 1970 official life tables.

We can examine the reliability of the Havana life tables and assess further the Cuban life tables by comparing the trends in life expectancy and the male-female differentials that they imply. Table 39 summarizes the trends in life expectancy at birth (e_0) for both sexes combined and by sex for Havana and Cuba; table 40 presents sex differentials in life expectancy for the same life tables.

We find certain anomalies when comparing the sex differentials in these tables. As the levels of life expectancy rise, the sex differentials widen, but with two deviations. The Havana life tables for 1901, at the very lowest levels of life expectancy, where the differentials generally are small, show a very wide gap between the sexes. This differential is suspicious; it is likely to have resulted from the unreliability of the data during that period or from the assumptions made in projecting the 1899 enumerated

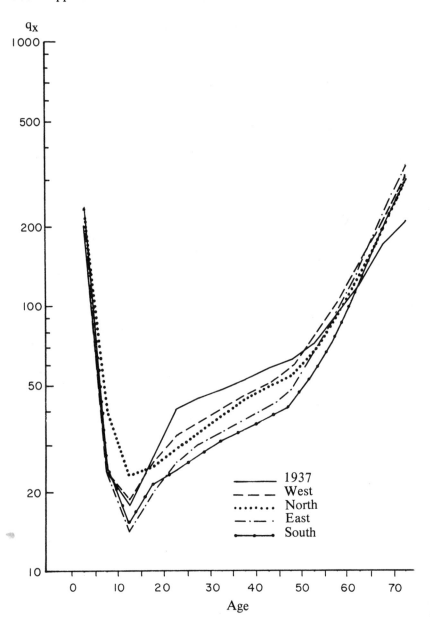

Figure 20. Female q_x Curves from 1937 Cuban Life Table and from Regional Model Life-Tables (Life Expectancy at Birth, 47.5 Years)

Table 39
Estimated Life Expectancy at Birth and Absolute and Average Yearly Gains

Estimated Life Expectancy at Birth						
Havana	1901	1907	1919	1931	1943	1953	
Both sexes	37.2	39.1	41.3	50.8	54.0	62.7	
Males	34.9	38.0	39.1	48.2	51.7	59.4	
Females	40.1	40.2	44.2	54.0	56.8	66.2	
Cuba		1905	1915	1925	1937	1953	1970
Both sexes		36.4	37.2	39.2	46.4	58.8	70.2
Males		35.7	36.5	38.4	44.8	56.7	68.5
Females		37.0	37.8	40.0	48.1	61.0	71.8

Absolute Yearly Gain					
Havana	1901-07	1907-19	1919-31	1931-43	1943-53
Both sexes	1.9	2.2	9.5	3.2	8.7
Males	3.1	1.1	9.1	3.5	7.7
Females	.1	4.0	9.8	2.8	9.4
Cuba	1905-15	1915-25	1925-37	1937-53	1953-70
Both sexes	.8	2.0	7.2	12.4	11.4
Males	.8	1.9	6.4	11.9	11.8
Females	.8	2.2	8.1	12.9	10.8

Average Yearly Gain					
Havana	1901-07	1907-19	1919-31	1931-43	1943-53
Both sexes	.32	.18	.79	.27	.87
Males	.52	.09	.76	.29	.77
Females	.02	.33	.82	.23	.94
Cuba	1905-15	1915-25	1925-37	1937-53	1953-70
Both sexes	.08	.20	.60	.78	.67
Males	.08	.19	.53	.74	.69
Females	.08	.22	.68	.81	.64

Table 40
Sex Differentials in Life Expectancy, Female over Male
(In Years)

Year	At Birth		At Exact Age Five	
	Havana	Cuba	Havana	Cuba
1901	5.2		4.1	
1905		1.3		.9
1907	2.2		1.3	
1915		1.3		.9
1919	5.1		4.9	
1925		1.6		1.6
1931	5.8		5.2	
1937		3.3		2.6
1943	5.1		5.0	
1953	6.8	4.3	6.5	3.2
1970		3.3		2.5

population to 1901 (which resulted in a distorted age distribution). Such large differentials contrast with the much smoother progression of the levels and sex differences in life expectancy observed in the later life-tables.

The 1907 Havana life tables, however, show a very narrow sex differential, which suggests some estimating biases. The biases are not likely to influence the interpretation of the trend, since it is apparent that only minor gains in life expectancy were made during the first years following the sanitary reforms instituted by the American occupation forces.

We see another significant deviation from the normal pattern in the 1970 life tables for Cuba, in which the gap between the sexes narrows substantially in comparison with the 1953 tables. This is puzzling, since it runs contrary to the established observation that at higher levels of life expectancy at birth, the sex differentials tend to increase.[9] This deviation makes suspect the quality of the data on which the 1970 life tables are based, though by every criterion, the tables appear to be exceptionally reliable. The possibility exists, therefore, that a true reversal may have occurred.

We should regard the very large gains in life expectancy for Havana between 1919 and 1931 with certain reservations. Although I do not question that large gains did in fact take place, I am not confident in accepting the estimated magnitude. There is some possibility that the life tables for Havana exaggerate the levels of life expectancy. A possible deterioration in the national death-registration system in the country at the time of the World Depression may lead to biased estimates. If so, there would be an overoptimistic representation of changes between 1919 and 1931, but an unduly pessimistic depiction of the changes between 1931 and 1943. This seems to be the case. However, the overall trend, in my view, remains unchanged, although the actual levels may vary. I base this interpretation on the analysis of death-by-cause statistics and other records.

We can observe a curious reversal of the e_x relation between the Havana and the Cuba series in figure 21. At age five the life expectancy levels for Cuba exceed or closely approximate those for Havana, which result contradicts what we might have expected, in view of the disparity in living conditions between Havana and the rest of the country. Furthermore, a similar reversal occurs at practically every age above ten. This anomaly may be explained in part by overestimation of the life-table mortality rates, but a more important influence appears to have been the registration of deaths in Havana by place of occurrence rather than by place of residence. Since the national health facilities of Cuba were heavily concentrated in the Havana area, many nonresidents of the city sought its superior facilities when stricken by disease, and many nonresidents died there. Figure 22 supports this argument. I chose 1953 to illustrate this argument partly because it is a recent year for which the data are relatively reliable, but primarily because it is the only year in which the time reference of the data is the same for Cuba and for Havana.

As figure 22 shows, the q_x values for Havana up to about age forty or forty-five lie below the corresponding values for Cuba. This is consistent with the postulated superior health conditions in Havana. However, after those ages, the q_x values for Havana exceed those of Cuba. This may have resulted because, at age forty or forty-five, when the incidence of degenerative diseases begins to increase rapidly, the number of deaths of nonresidents increased substantially, since their ailments could not be treated as successfully as the more easily treatable infectious diseases relatively more common at younger ages.

In summary, we can regard most of the life tables utilized in this study as valid, although some reservations are in order for others. In general, these life tables provide a description of the trend of mortality decline that is consistent with the trends shown by Andrew Collver's estimates of the secular trends of mortality in Cuba and by the rates I compiled for Havana obtained with crude and standardized rates.[10] This study's tables are also consistent with the life-table series estimated at the University of Havana for the first half of this century.[11]

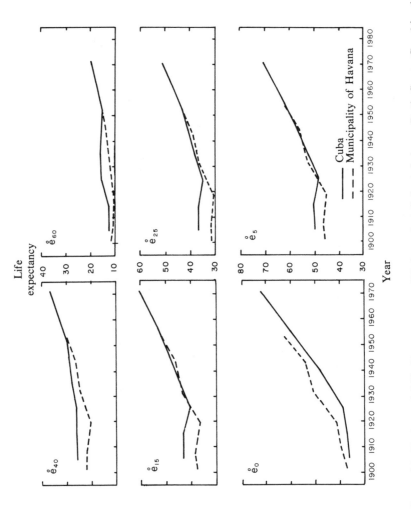

Figure 21. Estimated Life Expectancy at Birth and at Selected Ages, Both Sexes Combined

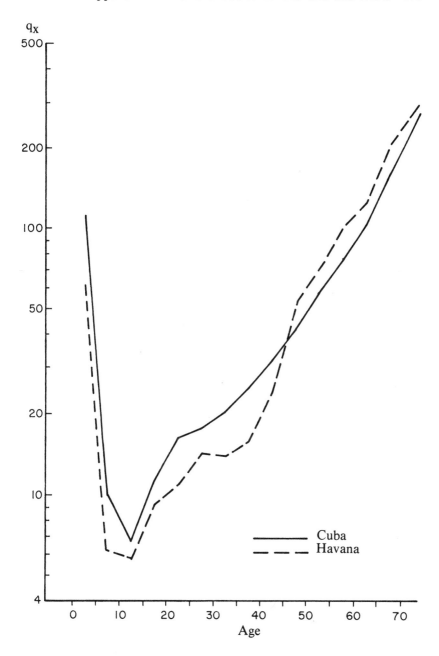

Figure 22. Life-Table Death Rates (q_x), Both Sexes Combined, 1953

Appendix 4: Classifications of Causes of Death

Since the data for Havana and Cuba on deaths by cause between 1901 and 1953 were coded according to the first six revisions of the International List of Causes of Death, it was necessary to group the data in order to make the secular series comparable. The grouping was also needed to reduce the number of categories to a manageable size.

The classificatory scheme used in this study was the one devised by Samuel Preston, Nathan Keyfitz, and Robert Schoen, which covers the second through seventh revisions of the International List of Causes of Death.[1] Eleven major categories are provided under this scheme: respiratory tuberculosis; other infectious and parasitic diseases; malignant and benign tumors; cardiovascular diseases; influenza, pneumonia, bronchitis; diarrhea, gastritis, enteritis; certain degenerative diseases; complications of pregnancy; certain diseases of infancy; accidents and violence; all other and unknown causes.

I had to derive a comparable classificatory grouping for the first revision, which, fortunately, is very similar to the second in its titles. Also I had to prepare the groupings for the sixth revision for the intermediate list. Preston et al. provided only the groupings for the sixth revision for the detailed and abridged lists.

I had to make some minor adjustments to the groupings given by Preston et al. They were required primarily because at times the Cuban data were not given with the needed detail. These adjustments do not affect very significantly the secular trends. They are described below by revisions.

Second Revision: Preston et al. placed title 61c (meningitis) among the "other infectious and parasitic diseases" and the remainder of 61 in the residual category. The data for Cuba are given only for 61, without further divisions. Hence, I decided to place 61 under "other infectious and parasitic diseases."

Third Revision: Preston et al. included title 91a under the "other infectious and parasitic diseases" (all of title 91 refers to diseases of the arteries). Titles 91b and 91c were placed under the cardiovascular diseases. I placed all of 91 under the cardiovascular diseases.

Fourth Revision: In the classification used by Preston et al., title 139a is found with the malignant and benign tumors. The balance of this title is in the residual category (the title refers to diseases of the female genital organs). In the grouping scheme I am using, I placed all of title 139 among the malignant and benign neoplasms.

Fifth Revision: Preston and his associates included under the "other infectious and parasitic diseases" titles 44a, 44c, and 44d (title 44 in the International List is also called "other infective and parasitic diseases"). The remainder of this title they located in the residual category. In this study all of title 44 appears under the "other infectious and parasitic diseases."

The minor titles (for more specific causes of death) that I used in this study for the analysis of the mortality trend by cause for Havana were abstracted from the six revisions of the International List of Causes of Death. I believe that these minor groupings of causes are not problematic, as they seem to be well defined from revision to revision. Two exceptions may be meningitis (particularly during the second revision and after the fourth). A separate category for whooping cough was not provided in the intermediate list for the sixth revision. Some of these difficulties are associated with refinements in the description of diseases and with changes in nomenclature. The numbers of the titles included under each of the major and minor categories from the first to the sixth revisions are given below. The titles for the minor groupings in the third revision are not included, since no data under this revision were used in the computation of cause-specific rates for Havana.

The specific revisions used in the computation of cause-specific mortality rates in each censal period in Havana were the following: first revision (1901); first revision (1907); second revision (1919); fourth revision (1931); fifth revision (1943); sixth revision (1953).

Some problems of comparability for specific causes of death within the "other infectious and parasitic" grouping are evident, particularly in 1901, 1943, and 1953. For these years the sum of the cause-specific rates shown exceeds the overall rate for the combined "other infectious and parasitic" grouping, because, as noted earlier, it was impossible to isolate with absolute certainty specific causes of death, such as meningitis, in certain revisions. Improvements in medical and nosological knowledge over time led to changes in the way in which causes of death were classified.

These classificatory difficulties in no way alter the conclusions of the study, although they do pose minor questions of uncertainty regarding the secular behavior of a few specific causes of death for the periods in which certain causes of death overlap from one major group of causes to another. The major groupings are not affected at all by these problems.

Major Groupings of Causes of Death in International List of Causes of Death

Respiratory tuberculosis

First Revision: code number, 27   Fourth Revision: 23
Second Revision: 28   Fifth Revision: 13
Third Revision: 31   Sixth Revision: 1

Other infectious and parasitic diseases

First Revision: code numbers, 1-9, 11-12, 14-23, 25-26, 28-30, 32-34, 36, 38, 61-62, 67, 72, 107, 111

Second Revision: 1-9, 11-12, 14-25, 29-35, 37-38, 61-62, 67, 106-107, 112, 164

Third Revision: 1-10, 12-14, 16-30, 32-42, 72, 76, 115-116, 121, 175

Fourth Revision: 1-10, 12-22, 24-44, 80, 83, 96, 177

Fifth Revision: 1-12, 14-32, 34-44, 177

Sixth Revision: 2-14, 16-18, 21-24, 28, 31-32, 36-37, 43

Malignant and benign tumors

First Revision: code numbers, 39-46, 53, 129, 131

Second Revision: 39-46, 53, 129, 131

Third Revision: 43-50, 65, 137, 139

Fourth Revision: 45-55, 72, 139

Fifth Revision: 45-57, 74

Sixth Revision: 44-60

Cardiovascular diseases

First Revision: code numbers, 47, 64-66, 77-86, 142

Second Revision: 47, 64-66, 77-85, 142

Third Revision: 51, 74-75, 83, 87-96, 151

Fourth Revision: 56, 82, 90-95, 97-103

Fifth Revision: 58, 83, 90-103

Sixth Revision: 70, 79-86

Influenza, pneumonia, bronchitis

First Revision: code numbers, 10, 90-93

Second Revision: 10, 89-92

Third Revision: 11, 99-101

Fourth Revision: 11, 106-109

Fifth Revision: 33, 106-109

Sixth Revision: 88-93

Diarrhea, gastritis, enteritis

First Revision: code numbers, 13, 105-106

Second Revision: 13, 104-105

Third Revision: 15, 113-114

Fourth Revision: 119-120

Fifth Revision: 119-120

Sixth Revision: 101, 104

Certain degenerative diseases (nephritis, cirrhosis of the liver, ulcers of stomach or duodenum, diabetes)

First Revision: code numbers, 50, 103, 112, 119-120

Second Revision: 50, 102, 113, 119-120

Third Revision: 57, 111, 122, 128-129

Fourth Revision: 59, 117, 124, 130-132

Fifth Revision: 61, 117, 124, 130-132

Sixth Revision: 63, 99-100, 105, 108-109

Complications of pregnancy

First Revision: code numbers, 134-141

Second Revision: 134-141

Third Revision: 143-150

Fourth Revision: 140-150

Fifth Revision: 140-150

Sixth Revision: 115-120

Certain diseases of infancy
First Revision: code numbers, 151-152
Second Revision: 151-152
Third Revision: 160-162
Fourth Revision: 158-161
Fifth Revision: 158-161
Sixth Revision: 130-135

Accidents and violence
First Revision: code numbers, 58, 153, 155-176
Second Revision: 58, 153, 155-163, 165-186
Third Revision: 67, 163, 165-174, 176-203
Fourth Revision: 77, 163-176, 178-198
Fifth Revision: 78, 163-176, 178-198
Sixth Revision: 138-150

All other and unknown causes
First Revision: code name, residual
Second Revision: Residual
Third Revision: Residual
Fourth Revision: Residual
Fifth Revision: Residual
Sixth Revision: Residual

Scarlet fever
First Revision: code number, 7
Second Revision: 7
Fourth Revision: 8
Fifth Revision: 8
Sixth Revision: 17

Whooping cough
First Revision: code number, 8
Second Revision: 8
Fourth Revision: 9
Fifth Revision: 9
Sixth Revision: No separate listing for whooping cough appeared in the intermediate International List of Causes of Death.

Measles
First Revision: code number, 6
Second Revision: 6
Fourth Revision: 7
Fifth Revision: 35
Sixth Revision: 32

Diphtheria
First Revision: code Number, 9
Second Revision: 9
Fourth Revision: 10
Fifth Revision: 10
Sixth Revision: 21

Dysentery
First Revision: code number, 14
Second Revision: 14
Fourth Revision: 13
Fifth Revision: 27
Sixth Revision: 16

Nonrespiratory tuberculosis
First Revision: code numbers, 26, 28-30, 32-34
Second Revision: 29-35
Fourth Revision: 24-32
Fifth Revision: 14-22
Sixth Revision: 2-5

Enteric fever (typhoid and paratyphoid fevers)

First Revision: code number, 1

Second Revision: 1

Fourth Revision: 1, 2

Fifth Revision: 1, 2

Sixth Revision: 12, 13

Malaria

First Revision: code number, 4

Second Revision: 4

Fourth Revision: 38

Fifth Revision: 28

Sixth Revision: 37

Syphilis

First Revision: code numbers, 36, 62, 67

Second Revision: 37, 62, 67

Fourth Revision: 34, 80, 83, 96

Fifth Revision: 30

Sixth Revision: 6-10

Meningitis

First Revision: code number, 61

Second Revision: 61

Fourth Revision: 18, 79

Fifth Revision: 6, 81

Sixth Revision: 23, 71

Tetanus

First Revision: code number, 72

Second Revision: 24

Fourth Revision: 22

Fifth Revision: 12

Sixth Revision: 26

Nephritis

First Revision: code numbers, 119-120

Second Revision: 119-120

Fourth Revision: 130-132

Fifth Revision: 130-132

Sixth Revision: 108-109

Old age

First Revision: code number, 154

Second Revision: 154

Fourth Revision: 162

Fifth Revision: 162

Sixth Revision: 136

Appendicitis, peritonitis

First Revision: code numbers, 116, 118

Second Revision: 108, 117

Fourth Revision: 121, 129

Fifth Revision: 121, 129

Sixth Revision: 102

Appendix 5: Statistical Appendix

Table 41
Estimated Crude Death Rates, City of Havana

Year	Rate	Year	Rate	Year	Rate
1880	39.9	1905	20.1	1930	14.0
1881	38.9	1906	20.7	1931	14.7
1882	32.2	1907	22.2	1932	14.4
1883	36.7	1908	19.5	1933	15.3
1884	32.9	1909	19.2	1934	15.1
1885	29.1	1910	19.9	1935	n.a.
1886	31.5	1911	19.3	1936	n.a.
1887	41.7	1912	18.3	1937	n.a.
1888	32.4	1913	18.8	1938	n.a.
1889	28.6	1914	19.4	1939	n.a.
1890	36.0	1915	18.8	1940	13.8
1891	33.8	1916	19.4	1941	n.a.
1892	33.2	1917	20.0	1942	n.a.
1893	30.3	1918	22.2	1943	14.3
1894	31.6	1919	21.0	1944	13.8
1895	32.3	1920	23.6	1945	14.2
1896	50.8	1921	19.0	1946	12.0
1897	77.1	1922	18.6	1947	11.5
1898	89.1	1923	16.6	1948	11.2
1899	33.7	1924	17.2	1949	11.5
1900	24.5	1925	17.3	1950	10.8
1901	22.4	1926	16.6	1951	11.2
1902	22.2	1927	17.4	1952	10.7
1903	19.7	1928	15.7	1953	10.7
1904	19.6	1929	15.2		

Source: Cuban censuses and vital statistics.

Note: n.a. means data not available.

Table 42
Life Tables, Municipality of Havana, 1901

	MALE					FEMALE				
Age	q_x	l_x	L_x	T_x	$e°_x$	q_x	l_x	L_x	T_x	$e°_x$
0	0.224533	100000	88773	3492746	34.927	0.188741	100000	89234	4007633	40.076
1-4	0.094725	77547	291823	3403974	43.896	0.081237	81126	308027	3918400	48.300
5-9	0.024634	70201	346682	3112152	44.332	0.023087	74535	368375	3610373	48.438
10-14	0.015092	68472	339985	2765470	40.388	0.018548	72815	360996	3241998	44.524
15-19	0.040551	67438	330873	2425485	35.966	0.044175	71464	349878	2881003	40.314
20-24	0.054358	64704	314887	2094613	32.372	0.051367	68307	333105	2531126	37.055
25-29	0.057313	61187	297305	1779727	29.087	0.073993	64798	312113	2198022	33.921
30-34	0.072511	57680	278261	1482423	25.701	0.067110	60004	289895	1885909	31.430
35-39	0.094032	53497	255138	1204163	22.509	0.080811	55977	268614	1596014	28.512
40-44	0.108771	48467	229604	949025	19.581	0.081865	51453	246888	1327400	25.798
45-49	0.166353	43195	198226	719421	16.655	0.111196	47241	223030	1080512	22.872
50-54	0.175004	36010	164072	521195	14.474	0.095432	41988	199896	857482	20.422
55-59	0.206166	29708	133317	357123	12.021	0.134848	37981	177211	657586	17.314
60-64	0.285575	23583	101156	223806	9.490	0.137995	32859	153516	480376	14.619
65-69	0.385665	16848	67779	122650	7.280	0.274875	28325	122392	326860	11.540
70-74	0.549571	10350	36894	54871	5.301	0.275014	20539	88306	204467	9.955
75-79	0.737679	4662	13710	17977	3.856	0.436326	14891	57741	116162	7.801
80-84	0.716089	1223	3279	4267	3.489	0.404969	8393	32801	58420	6.960
85+	1.000000	347	988	988	2.846	1.000000	4994	25619	25619	5.130

Source: Cuban censuses and vital statistics.

Table 43
Life Tables, Municipality of Havana, 1907

Age	MALE					FEMALE				
	q_x	l_x	L_x	T_x	e^o_x	q_x	l_x	L_x	T_x	e^o_x
0	0.182836	100000	89356	3801039	38.010	0.156489	100000	90069	4021379	40.214
1-4	0.092833	81716	307901	3711683	45.421	0.093229	84351	317744	3931311	46.607
5-9	0.027603	74130	365537	3403783	45.916	0.026433	76487	377381	3613567	47.244
10-14	0.020629	72084	356787	3038247	42.149	0.019677	74465	368910	3236186	43.459
15-19	0.034622	70597	347191	2681461	37.983	0.043879	73000	357376	2867277	39.278
20-24	0.044046	68153	333474	2334270	34.250	0.047373	69797	341068	2509901	35.960
25-29	0.053248	65151	317199	2000797	30.710	0.071261	66490	320767	2168863	32.619
30-34	0.057701	61682	299658	1683599	27.295	0.066040	61752	298505	1848096	29.928
35-39	0.071768	58123	280506	1383941	23.811	0.077119	57674	277262	1549591	26.868
40-44	0.094503	53951	257460	1103435	20.452	0.077635	53226	255906	1272329	23.904
45-49	0.131474	48853	228635	845956	17.316	0.100853	49094	233205	1016423	20.704
50-54	0.168508	42430	194438	617321	14.549	0.105913	44143	209282	783218	17.743
55-59	0.204201	35280	158725	422883	11.986	0.156608	39468	182351	573936	14.542
60-64	0.311874	28076	118642	264157	9.409	0.207676	33287	149621	391585	11.764
65-69	0.410838	19320	76071	145515	7.532	0.319840	26374	110819	241964	9.174
70-74	0.480632	11383	42353	69444	6.101	0.395781	17938	71481	131145	7.311
75-79	0.626094	5912	19508	27091	4.583	0.573739	10839	37711	59664	5.505
80-84	0.743474	2210	6295	7583	3.431	0.564097	4620	15666	21953	4.752
85+	1.000000	567	1288	1288	2.271	1.000000	2014	6287	6287	3.122

Source: Cuban censuses and vital statistics.

Table 44
Life Tables, Municipality of Havana, 1919

Age	MALE q_x	l_x	L_x	T_x	e^o_x	FEMALE q_x	l_x	L_x	T_x	e^o_x
0	0.119808	100000	91524	3914680	39.147	0.101499	100000	92455	4415568	44.156
1-4	0.077809	88019	334955	3823156	43.435	0.074825	89850	342593	4323114	48.115
5-9	0.023128	81171	401160	3488201	42.974	0.021993	83127	411065	3980522	47.885
10-14	0.017650	79293	393253	3087042	38.932	0.016082	81299	403503	3569458	43.905
15-19	0.041709	77894	382070	2693789	34.583	0.039543	79991	392589	3165955	39.579
20-24	0.065267	74645	361298	2311720	30.970	0.050777	76828	374642	2773366	36.098
25-29	0.063990	69773	337704	1950423	27.954	0.060080	72927	353843	2398724	32.892
30-34	0.074654	65308	314586	1612720	24.694	0.068220	68546	331172	2044881	29.832
35-39	0.092423	60433	288632	1298135	21.481	0.078694	63869	306810	1713709	26.831
40-44	0.126680	54847	257384	1009503	18.406	0.081724	58843	282309	1406900	23.909
45-49	0.168489	47899	219604	752119	15.702	0.103232	54034	256349	1124591	20.812
50-54	0.208610	39829	178315	532515	13.370	0.111344	48456	229070	868243	17.918
55-59	0.247381	31520	137987	354200	11.237	0.160376	43061	198473	639173	14.843
60-64	0.326066	23723	99065	216213	9.114	0.206693	36155	162376	440700	12.189
65-69	0.424445	15988	62366	117148	7.327	0.288133	28682	122829	278324	9.704
70-74	0.508499	9202	33480	54812	5.957	0.384753	20418	81111	155495	7.616
75-79	0.618513	4523	14903	21332	4.717	0.528495	12562	45301	73384	5.842
80-84	0.716060	1725	5053	6429	3.726	0.587592	5923	19973	28083	4.741
85+	1.000000	490	1377	1377	2.810	1.000000	2443	8110	8110	3.320

Source: Cuban censuses and vital statistics.

Table 45
Life Tables, Municipality of Havana, 1931

Age	MALE					FEMALE				
	q_x	l_x	L_x	T_x	e_x^o	q_x	l_x	L_x	T_x	e_x^o
0	0.088090	100000	93223	4821583	48.216	0.068388	100000	94481	5400894	54.009
1-4	0.045869	91191	354307	4728361	51.851	0.043660	93161	362476	5306413	56.959
5-9	0.015614	87008	431644	4374055	50.272	0.011848	89094	442830	4943937	55.491
10-14	0.011421	85650	425968	3942411	46.030	0.009782	88038	438317	4501107	51.127
15-19	0.025415	84671	418274	3516444	41.530	0.027467	87177	430290	4062790	46.604
20-24	0.029136	82519	406706	3098170	37.545	0.032320	84783	417087	3632500	42.845
25-29	0.034058	80115	393911	2691464	33.595	0.030655	82042	403891	3215413	39.192
30-34	0.040796	77387	379280	2297554	29.689	0.032431	79527	391366	2811523	35.353
35-39	0.052281	74230	361907	1918274	25.842	0.043763	76948	376512	2420157	31.452
40-44	0.076389	70349	338882	1556367	22.124	0.047418	73581	359380	2043646	27.774
45-49	0.102067	64975	308888	1217486	18.738	0.061665	70092	340137	1684267	24.029
50-54	0.140928	58343	271982	908599	15.573	0.088399	65769	315072	1344131	20.437
55-59	0.211066	50121	224616	636617	12.702	0.132951	59956	280331	1029059	17.164
60-64	0.263618	39542	171566	412001	10.419	0.156336	51984	240021	748728	14.403
65-69	0.349365	29118	120059	240435	8.257	0.227362	43857	194785	508707	11.599
70-74	0.525166	18945	68540	120376	6.354	0.300390	33886	143933	313921	9.264
75-79	0.430566	8996	34059	51836	5.762	0.410737	23707	93549	169988	7.170
80-84	0.783477	5123	15003	17776	3.470	0.508164	13970	51235	76439	5.472
85+	1.000000	1109	2773	2773	2.500	1.000000	6871	25204	25204	3.668

Source: Cuban censuses and vital statistics.

Table 46
Life Tables, Municipality of Havana, 1943

Age	MALE					FEMALE				
	q_x	l_x	L_x	T_x	e^o_x	q_x	l_x	L_x	T_x	e^o_x
0	0.077313	100000	93892	5173801	51.738	0.068128	100000	94499	5677136	56.771
1-4	0.041716	92269	359452	5079909	55.056	0.040318	93187	363356	5582637	59.908
5-9	0.012221	88420	439397	4720457	53.387	0.011661	89430	444543	5219282	58.362
10-14	0.011873	87339	434280	4281061	49.017	0.010826	88387	439733	4774739	54.021
15-19	0.022368	86302	426866	3846782	44.573	0.022326	87430	432545	4335006	49.582
20-24	0.022648	84372	417149	3419916	40.534	0.026570	85478	421760	3902461	45.654
25-29	0.027322	82461	406789	3002768	36.414	0.026103	83207	410633	3480702	41.832
30-34	0.030823	80208	395003	2595980	32.366	0.029645	81035	399229	3070069	37.886
35-39	0.037880	77736	381899	2200978	28.314	0.031173	78633	387174	2670841	33.966
40-44	0.070456	74791	361394	1819079	24.322	0.040187	76182	373540	2283667	29.977
45-49	0.084682	69522	333259	1457685	20.957	0.052210	73120	356544	1910128	26.123
50-54	0.110672	63634	301237	1124426	17.670	0.077881	69303	333694	1553584	22.417
55-59	0.161023	56592	261104	823189	14.546	0.110345	63905	302362	1219891	19.089
60-64	0.241937	47479	208971	562086	11.839	0.134177	56854	265561	917529	16.138
65-69	0.292123	35992	153385	353115	9.811	0.175787	49225	224985	651998	13.245
70-74	0.396082	25478	101335	199730	7.839	0.246153	40572	178322	427014	10.525
75-79	0.425222	15387	59674	98396	6.395	0.350314	30585	125924	248691	8.131
80-84	0.651291	8844	29029	38721	4.378	0.450559	19871	76423	122767	6.178
85+	1.000000	3084	9692	9692	3.143	1.000000	10918	46344	46344	4.245

Source: Cuban censuses and vital statistics.

Table 47
Life Tables, Municipality of Havana, 1953

Age	MALE					FEMALE				
	q_x	l_x	L_x	T_x	e^o_x	q_x	l_x	L_x	T_x	e^o_x
0	0.056439	100000	95319	5935339	59.353	0.039691	100000	96586	6662374	66.624
1-4	0.014731	94356	373949	5840020	61.893	0.013767	96031	380818	6565789	68.372
5-9	0.007136	92966	463172	5466071	58.796	0.005270	94709	472296	6184971	65.305
10-14	0.006863	92303	459989	5002899	54.201	0.004734	94210	469991	5712675	60.638
15-19	0.010349	91669	456060	4542910	49.558	0.008285	93764	466986	5242684	55.914
20-24	0.011491	90721	451082	4086851	45.049	0.010461	92987	462600	4775699	51.359
25-29	0.015166	89678	445071	3635769	40.542	0.013562	92014	456985	4313099	46.874
30-34	0.016175	88318	438093	3190699	36.127	0.012550	90766	450969	3856114	42.484
35-39	0.019726	86890	430462	2752607	31.679	0.013196	89627	445251	3405145	37.992
40-44	0.033639	85176	419576	2322146	27.263	0.016808	88444	438907	2959895	33.466
45-49	0.071071	82310	397721	1902570	23.115	0.035808	86958	427631	2520988	28.991
50-54	0.087299	76460	366250	1504850	19.681	0.053598	83844	408597	2093358	24.967
55-59	0.127491	69786	327469	1138601	16.316	0.076247	79350	381978	1684762	21.232
60-64	0.169118	60838	279628	811162	13.322	0.084439	73300	351955	1302785	17.773
65-69	0.264024	50591	220154	531534	10.506	0.156582	67111	310582	950831	14.168
70-74	0.352778	37234	152805	311381	8.363	0.219634	56602	252614	640249	11.311
75-79	0.449447	24099	92268	158576	6.580	0.312024	44170	186462	387635	8.776
80-84	0.574953	13268	45979	66308	4.998	0.419517	30388	119773	201173	6.620
85+	1.000000	5639	20329	20329	3.605	1.000000	17640	81400	81400	4.615

Source: Cuban censuses and vital statistics.

Table 48
Life Tables, Cuba, 1919-1931

Age	MALE					FEMALE				
	q_x	l_x	L_x	T_x	e_x^o	q_x	l_x	L_x	T_x	e_x^o
0-4	0.27279	100000	392935	3836401	38.36	0.26510	100000	395905	3995368	39.95
5-9	0.03642	72721	357471	3443466	47.35	0.03376	73490	361707	3599463	48.98
10-14	0.02501	70072	346312	3085996	44.04	0.02608	71099	350763	3237757	45.60
15-19	0.03946	68320	335351	2739685	40.10	0.04221	69157	339016	2886995	41.75
20-24	0.05842	65624	319202	2404334	36.64	0.05927	66238	322057	2547980	38.47
25-29	0.06384	61790	299765	2085132	33.75	0.06610	62312	301966	2225924	35.72
30-34	0.06821	57845	280031	1785367	30.86	0.07013	58193	281452	1923959	33.06
35-39	0.07568	53899	259978	1505336	27.93	0.07507	54112	261081	1642507	30.35
40-44	0.08885	49820	238746	1245358	25.00	0.07976	50050	240925	1381426	27.60
45-49	0.10636	45394	215634	1006613	22.18	0.08949	46057	220643	1140502	24.76
50-54	0.12860	40566	190526	790978	19.50	0.10473	41936	199371	919859	21.93
55-59	0.15675	35349	163601	600452	16.99	0.12396	37544	176753	720489	19.19
60-64	0.18891	29808	135589	426852	14.66	0.15239	32890	152570	543736	16.53
65-69	0.22587	24177	107732	301263	12.46	0.17879	27878	127509	391167	14.03
70-74	0.27682	18716	80953	193530	10.34	0.21710	22894	102520	263658	11.52
75+	1.00000	13535	112577	112577	8.32	1.00000	17923	161138	161138	8.99

Source: Rodolfo Mezquita, *Cuba: Estimación de la mortalidad por sexo. Tabla de vida para los períodos 1919-1931 y 1931-1943*, series C, no. 121 (Santiago, Chile: Centro Latinoamericano de Demografía, March 1970), p. 33-34.

Table 49
Life Tables, Cuba, 1931-1943

Age	MALE q_x	l_x	L_x	T_x	$e°_x$	FEMALE q_x	l_x	L_x	T_x	$e°_x$
0-4	0.22274	100000	413810	4475726	44.76	0.20119	100000	425010	4807193	48.07
5-9	0.02379	77726	384358	4061916	52.26	0.02383	79881	395007	4382183	54.86
10-14	0.01623	75877	376546	2677558	48.47	0.01790	77977	386664	3987177	51.13
15-19	0.02779	74646	368434	3301013	44.22	0.02696	76581	378133	3600513	47.02
20-24	0.04269	72572	355675	2932580	40.41	0.04067	74517	365559	3222380	43.24
25-29	0.04624	69474	339916	2576906	37.09	0.04509	71486	349954	2856821	39.96
30-34	0.05120	66261	323428	2236991	33.76	0.04906	68263	333541	2506867	36.72
35-39	0.05870	62869	305760	1913564	30.44	0.05539	64914	316519	2173326	33.48
40-44	0.07069	59178	286138	1607804	27.17	0.05823	61448	298921	1856808	30.22
45-49	0.08235	54995	264392	1321666	24.03	0.06262	57870	280916	1557888	26.92
50-54	0.09785	50466	240755	1057275	20.95	0.07307	54246	261987	1276972	23.54
55-59	0.12299	45528	214449	816521	17.93	0.09548	50283	240166	1014985	20.19
60-64	0.16335	39929	184147	602072	15.08	0.12250	45482	214285	774819	17.04
65-69	0.21518	33406	149758	417924	12.51	0.17134	39910	183278	560535	14.04
70-74	0.25972	26218	114559	268166	10.23	0.20973	33072	148715	377257	11.41
75+	1.00000	19408	153607	153607	7.91	1.00000	26136	228542	228542	8.74

Source: Rodolfo Mezquita, *Cuba: Estimación de la mortalidad por sexo. Tabla de vida para los períodos 1919-1931 y 1931-1943*, series C, no. 121 (Santiago, Chile: Centro Latinoamericano de Demografía, March 1970), pp. 33-34.

Table 50
Life Tables, Cuba, 1952-1954

Age	MALE					FEMALE				
	q_x	l_x	L_x	T_x	e^o_x	q_x	l_x	L_x	T_x	e^o_x
0	0.09069	100000	93652	5668625	56.69	0.06960	100000	95128	6100867	61.01
1	0.01718	90931	90009	5574973	61.31	0.01587	93040	92169	6005739	64.55
2-4	0.01967	89369	265559	5484964	61.37	0.01832	91563	272240	5913570	64.58
5-9	0.01035	87611	436058	5219405	59.57	0.00951	89886	447644	5641330	62.76
10-14	0.00673	86704	431852	4783347	55.17	0.00663	89031	443609	5193686	58.34
15-19	0.01208	86121	428395	4351495	50.53	0.01075	88441	439815	4750077	53.71
20-24	0.01829	85080	421680	3923100	46.11	0.01470	87491	434459	4310262	49.27
25-29	0.02001	83524	413861	3501420	41.92	0.01618	86205	427914	3875803	44.96
30-34	0.02246	81852	405066	3087559	37.72	0.01908	84810	420260	3447889	40.65
35-39	0.02803	80013	394894	2682493	33.53	0.02300	83192	411613	3027629	36.39
40-44	0.03662	77770	382282	2287599	29.41	0.02764	81278	401250	2616016	32.19
45-49	0.04953	74922	365976	1905317	25.43	0.03347	79031	388971	2214766	28.02
50-54	0.06779	71211	344786	1539341	21.62	0.04552	76386	373871	1825795	23.90
55-59	0.09096	66384	317790	1194555	17.99	0.06064	72909	354247	1451924	19.91
60-64	0.12241	60346	284334	876765	14.53	0.08378	68488	329014	1097677	16.03
65-69	0.17917	52959	242164	592431	11.19	0.13798	62750	293293	768663	12.25
70-74	0.28662	43471	186919	350267	8.06	0.23908	54092	239216	475370	8.79
75-79	0.54512	31011	110584	163348	5.27	0.49408	41160	153190	236154	5.74
80-84	0.69968	14106	42913	52764	3.74	0.66516	20824	65957	82964	3.98
85+	1.00000	4236	9851	9851	2.33	1.00000	6973	17007	17007	2.44

Source: Fernando González Q. and Jorge Debasa, *Cuba: Evaluación y ajuste del censo de 1953 y las estadísticas de nacimientos y defunciones entre 1943 y 1958. Tabla de mortalidad por sexo, 1952-54*, series C, no. 124 (Santiago, Chile: Centro Latinoamericano de Demografía, 1970), p. 27.

Table 51
Life Tables, Cuba, 1970

Age	MALE q_x	l_x	L_x	T_x	e°_x	FEMALE q_x	l_x	L_x	T_x	e°_x
0	0.051180	100000	95727	6846471	68.5	0.039674	100000	96728	7175880	71.8
1	0.002778	94882	94727	6750744	71.1	0.002718	96032	95877	7079152	73.7
2	0.001489	94818	94542	6656017	70.3	0.001390	95771	95701	6983275	72.9
3	0.001090	94477	94473	6561475	69.5	0.001020	95639	95588	6887574	72.0
4	0.000590	94374	94341	6467052	68.5	0.000600	95541	95512	6791986	71.1
5–9	0.002647	94309	471698	6372711	67.8	0.002098	95484	476190	6696474	70.1
10–14	0.003096	94059	469355	5901013	62.7	0.002547	95284	475471	6220284	65.3
15–19	0.006232	93768	467200	5431858	57.9	0.004541	95041	474725	5744813	60.4
20–24	0.007375	93184	464189	4964458	53.3	0.005437	94609	471560	5270088	55.7
25–29	0.008021	92497	460870	4500269	48.7	0.006083	94095	468852	4798528	51.0
30–34	0.009161	91755	457065	4039399	44.0	0.007226	93523	466207	4329676	46.3
35–39	0.011440	90914	452174	3582334	39.4	0.009706	92847	462051	3863469	41.6
40–44	0.015242	89874	446254	3130160	34.8	0.013269	91946	456929	3401418	37.0
45–49	0.021877	88504	438009	2683906	30.3	0.018393	90726	449865	2944489	32.5
50–54	0.032455	86568	428404	2245897	25.9	0.026667	89057	439815	2494624	28.0
55–59	0.049725	83758	409136	1819493	21.7	0.040380	86682	425273	2054809	23.7
60–64	0.079347	79593	385192	1410357	17.7	0.063233	83182	403684	1629536	19.6
65–69	0.129345	73278	344029	1027165	14.0	0.103289	77922	370705	1225852	15.7
70–74	0.210973	63800	286688	683186	10.7	0.167503	69874	321538	855147	12.2
75–79	0.328991	50340	209484	396448	7.9	0.276300	58170	251676	523609	9.2
80–84	0.548378	33275	118837	186984	5.6	0.444775	42098	162775	281933	6.7
85+	1.000000	15194	68147	68147	4.5	1.000000	23374	119158	119158	5.1

Source: Junta Central de Planificación, *La esperanza o expectativa de vida*, (Havana, 1974).

Table 52
Absolute Number of Deaths by Selected Causes, City of Havana

	Yellow Fever	Smallpox	Malaria	Diphtheria	Infantile Tetanus	Typhoid	Tuberculosis	All Deaths
1880	645	446	335	64	340	159	1,629	7,942
1881	485	706	228	77	379	322	1,679	7,767
1882	729	1	191	33	319	132	1,427	6,433
1883	849	5	183	52	310	154	1,471	7,341
1884	511	1	196	38	306	174	1,497	6,586
1885	165	0	101	32	198	115	1,239	5,823
1886	167	0	135	22	189	111	1,187	6,316
1887	532	1,654	269	137	335	176	1,527	8,362
1888	468	550	208	128	363	152	1,326	6,605
1889	303	7	228	103	343	178	1,382	5,923
1890	308	12	170	105	355	183	1,606	7,599
1891	356	151	203	78	320	154	1,563	7,249
1892	357	0	202	84	256	366	1,528	7,221
1893	496	8	240	147	282	208	1,342	6,697
1894	382	216	201	76	173	100	1,314	7,101
1895	553	181	206	25	180	183	1,623	7,362
1896	1,282	1,004	450	19	232	487	1,578	11,762
1897	858	1,404	811	36	215	679	1,926	18,135
1898	136	168	1,907	23	173	1,012	2,794	21,252
1899	103	4	909	39	92	140	981	8,153
1900	310	2	344	15	139	90	851	6,102
1901	18	0	151	25	128	83	900	5,720
1902	0	0	77	25	68	87	949	5,832

Source: Cuban vital statistics.

Table 53
Age-Sex-Standardized Cause-Specific Death Rates,
Municipality of Havana

	1907	1919	1931
Respiratory tuberculosis	379.0	344.3	164.6
Other infectious and parasitic diseases	236.7	125.9	59.8
Malignant and benign tumors	139.0	186.9	147.9
Cardiovascular diseases	779.4	760.6	537.6
Influenza, pneumonia, bronchitis	188.1	175.8	152.5
Diarrhea, gastritis, enteritis	207.6	273.6	160.2
Certain degenerative diseases	113.0	173.6	144.1
Complications of pregnancy	20.4	23.0	14.4
Certain diseases of infancy	69.8	42.5	24.7
Accidents and violence	81.8	101.8	97.7
All other and unknown causes	311.3	241.8	246.6
All causes	2,526.1	2,449.8	1,750.0

Notes: The rates have been standardized to the age-sex structure of the 1943 population. All rates are shown per 100,000 population.

Rates computed with unadjusted population for underenumeration of children under one year of age.

Table 54
Absolute Number of Deaths by Groups of Causes, Municipality of Havana

	I	II	III	IV	V	VI	VII	VIII	IX	X	XI	Total
1902	885	918	201	1,235	516	703	278	60	216	222	598	5,832
1903	969	897	229	1,221	413	353	266	47	205	183	699	5,482
1904	1,071	837	221	1,101	430	485	259	70	235	183	691	5,583
1905	1,073	785	256	1,184	475	571	265	41	226	187	768	5,831
1906	1,032	696	282	1,440	477	577	307	49	249	266	769	6,144
1907	1,041	870	291	1,520	595	761	262	57	272	240	799	6,708
1908	1,079	549	343	1,372	471	727	262	58	214	234	685	5,994
1909	911	633	360	1,321	522	738	287	64	211	274	676	5,997
1910	1,006	572	369	1,501	507	935	279	55	231	215	661	6,331
1911	1,056	629	367	1,388	502	934	288	61	186	199	617	6,227
1912	976	577	359	1,425	384	871	329	62	188	247	586	6,004
1913	935	615	376	1,599	371	883	342	47	186	248	662	6,264
1914	1,023	609	425	1,716	345	983	358	64	164	278	605	6,570
1915	1,005	633	391	1,646	430	767	350	70	190	268	716	6,466
1916	1,049	496	407	1,750	511	891	415	66	224	274	676	6,759
1917	1,106	478	449	1,786	552	989	421	72	200	293	712	7,058
1918	1,294	517	430	1,889	1,043	1,027	404	60	203	304	771	7,942
1919	1,135	480	494	1,916	619	1,119	490	77	190	350	759	7,629
1920	1,137	628	445	2,272	781	1,522	538	80	211	382	920	8,916
1921	1,035	405	428	1,879	552	1,098	511	74	193	381	901	7,457
1922	1,027	404	450	1,833	560	1,396	464	69	186	365	839	7,593
1923	882	322	511	1,826	511	960	518	59	169	352	895	7,005
1924	975	420	495	1,879	612	1,020	519	75	169	368	1,005	7,537

Groups of Causes

Table 54—Continued

| | | | | | | Groups of Causes | | | | | | |
	I	II	III	IV	V	VI	VII	VIII	IX	X	XI	Total
1925	1,062	353	580	1,929	650	1,103	496	80	151	400	1,042	7,846
1926	1,003	397	542	1,770	609	1,123	527	83	160	428	1,144	7,786
1927	1,012	350	604	2,200	671	1,128	630	88	167	397	1,172	8,419
1928	856	351	595	2,025	635	937	574	65	139	430	1,196	7,803
1929	852	386	546	1,936	684	876	604	66	153	437	1,251	7,791
1930	834	259	653	1,983	619	699	590	60	128	423	1,159	7,407
1931	828	314	625	2,182	743	825	633	73	124	499	1,142	7,988
1932	795	303	601	2,149	736	860	672	63	208	433	1,168	7,988
1933	964	336	636	2,318	879	847	655	60	176	667	1,096	8,634
1934	863	474	641	2,386	872	808	739	78	150	521	1,141	8,673
1935	n.a.	n.a.	n.a.	n.a.	n.a.	n.a.	n.a.	n.a.	n.a.	n.a.	n.a.	n.a.
1936	n.a.	n.a.	n.a.	n.a.	n.a.	n.a.	n.a.	n.a.	n.a.	n.a.	n.a.	n.a.
1937	n.a.	n.a.	n.a.	n.a.	n.a.	n.a.	n.a.	n.a.	n.a.	n.a.	n.a.	n.a.
1938	n.a.	n.a.	n.a.	n.a.	n.a.	n.a.	n.a.	n.a.	n.a.	n.a.	n.a.	n.a.
1939	n.a.	n.a.	n.a.	n.a.	n.a.	n.a.	n.a.	n.a.	n.a.	n.a.	n.a.	n.a.
1940	1,004	424	1,026	2,325	867	577	634	67	149	414	1,358	8,845
1941	n.a.	n.a.	n.a.	n.a.	n.a.	n.a.	n.a.	n.a.	n.a.	n.a.	n.a.	n.a.
1942	n.a.	n.a.	n.a.	n.a.	n.a.	n.a.	n.a.	n.a.	n.a.	n.a.	n.a.	n.a.
1943	1,197	506	1,151	2,748	764	558	681	44	142	407	1,502	9,700
1944	1,098	469	1,210	2,709	695	479	689	54	143	442	1,472	9,460
1945	1,103	433	1,237	2,984	632	617	625	42	142	503	1,612	9,930
1946	990	338	1,182	2,699	487	265	549	41	124	486	1,392	8,553
1947	969	293	1,275	2,553	480	214	519	41	115	510	1,340	8,309
1948	755	254	1,340	2,710	390	237	583	28	104	518	1,275	8,194
1949	733	236	1,386	2,918	376	226	601	34	144	541	1,330	8,525

Table 54—*Continued*

Groups of Causes

	I	II	III	IV	V	VI	VII	VIII	IX	X	XI	Total
1950	699	146	1,434	3,022	317	77	467	23	120	470	1,383	8,158
1951	702	149	1,442	3,173	362	289	562	27	165	480	1,214	8,565
1952	497	118	1,622	3,210	281	161	560	20	189	513	1,135	8,306
1953	340	90	1,609	3,309	299	188	579	14	199	468	1,327	8,422

Source: Cuban vital statistics.

Note: I = respiratory tuberculosis; II=other infectious and parasitic diseases; III =malignant and benign tumors; IV=cardiovascular diseases; V=influenza, pneumonia, and bronchitis; VI=diarrhea, gastritis, and enteritis; VII=certain degenerative diseases; VIII=complications of pregnancy; IX=certain diseases of infancy; X=accidents and violence; XI=all other and unknown causes.

n.a. means data not available.

Table 55

Absolute Number of Deaths by Groups of Causes, Cuba

	I	II	III	IV	V	VI	VII	VIII	IX	X	XI	Total
						Groups of Causes						
1902	3,602	5,671	581	3,749	1,880	3,227	933	337	546	967	3,989	25,482
1903	3,440	5,249	644	3,637	1,789	2,592	949	322	753	948	3,659	23,982
1904	3,545	5,160	718	3,562	2,101	3,146	970	385	1,061	935	3,615	25,198
1905	3,609	5,189	816	3,905	2,151	4,321	1,061	415	1,224	1,077	3,577	27,345
1906	3,560	5,110	877	4,400	2,549	4,949	1,154	501	1,538	1,367	4,017	30,022
1907	3,578	5,083	881	5,187	2,824	7,650	1,254	481	1,568	1,220	4,274	34,000
1908	3,129	4,197	970	4,443	2,515	5,525	1,110	423	1,255	1,228	3,548	28,343
1909	2,877	4,136	1,053	4,487	2,752	5,455	1,222	468	1,356	1,329	3,697	28,832
1910	3,032	3,810	1,065	5,432	3,591	7,879	1,410	469	1,744	1,351	4,061	33,844
1911	3,156	3,621	1,086	5,162	2,946	7,556	1,431	479	1,532	1,234	3,854	32,057
1912	2,898	3,348	1,091	4,994	2,691	7,018	1,425	493	1,446	1,560	3,915	30,879
1913	2,943	3,493	1,227	5,623	3,114	7,587	1,492	537	1,479	1,490	4,308	33,293
1914	3,157	3,921	1,294	6,109	3,227	8,359	1,696	520	1,631	1,512	4,495	35,921
1915	3,194	3,680	1,311	6,367	3,316	7,289	1,676	550	1,466	1,515	4,711	35,075
1916	3,343	3,801	1,378	7,050	3,886	10,658	1,998	518	1,762	1,538	5,010	40,942
1917	3,269	3,657	1,349	7,135	4,019	9,462	2,018	514	1,706	1,932	4,791	39,902
1918	3,901	3,937	1,474	7,253	9,800	8,914	2,147	620	1,552	1,778	4,838	46,214
1919	3,558	3,379	1,502	7,391	5,051	9,324	2,195	622	1,539	1,835	4,781	41,177
1920	3,866	4,932	1,518	8,666	5,973	13,142	2,628	646	1,910	2,037	5,729	51,047
1921	3,473	5,084	1,504	7,829	4,716	11,014	2,477	594	1,803	2,126	6,017	46,637
1922	3,369	3,641	1,556	7,767	4,174	11,223	2,443	591	1,646	1,887	5,374	43,671
1923	3,112	3,052	1,678	7,707	4,613	9,629	2,545	500	1,594	1,827	5,659	41,916
1924	3,220	3,188	1,733	7,830	4,766	9,857	2,510	527	1,687	1,890	5,609	42,817

Table 55—Continued

	I	II	III	IV	V	VI	VII	VIII	IX	X	XI	Total
						Groups of Causes						
1925	3,287	3,096	1,869	8,063	4,739	9,349	2,588	550	1,528	1,986	5,787	42,842
1926	3,279	3,536	1,960	8,507	4,727	10,375	2,732	561	1,546	2,163	5,966	45,352
1927	3,302	3,073	1,905	9,651	4,915	10,770	2,970	559	1,628	1,947	6,147	46,867
1928	2,942	2,604	1,849	8,775	4,890	7,396	2,741	481	1,462	2,083	5,748	40,971
1929	2,948	2,726	1,686	8,705	4,890	8,444	2,793	533	1,552	2,049	5,847	42,173
1930	2,906	2,247	1,828	8,676	4,146	6,246	2,730	466	1,377	2,118	5,178	37,918
1931	2,836	2,309	1,796	9,319	4,669	6,868	2,925	509	1,392	2,353	5,460	40,436
1932	2,843	2,786	1,832	9,518	5,332	7,380	3,275	579	1,320	2,553	5,937	43,355
1933	3,236	3,888	1,797	10,545	6,216	9,375	3,588	501	1,414	2,584	7,087	50,231
1934	2,856	4,695	1,998	10,726	5,852	7,497	3,639	513	1,380	2,222	6,772	48,150
1935	2,884	3,765	2,066	9,952	7,799	9,057	3,391	466	1,779	2,160	6,581	49,900
1936	2,943	3,001	2,176	9,686	6,517	7,491	3,138	459	1,641	2,041	5,799	44,892
1937	2,601	2,597	2,332	8,925	6,304	7,451	2,989	348	1,470	1,959	5,854	42,830
1938	2,725	2,652	2,383	9,833	6,203	8,441	2,966	460	1,532	1,708	6,135	45,038
1939	2,658	2,402	2,810	9,981	6,653	6,622	2,935	423	1,625	1,828	6,252	44,189
1940	2,833	2,519	2,633	9,918	6,032	6,307	2,922	446	1,631	1,950	6,272	43,463
1941	n.a.	n.a.	n.a.	n.a.	n.a.	n.a.	n.a.	n.a.	n.a.	n.a.	n.a.	n.a.
1942	n.a.	n.a.	n.a.	n.a.	n.a.	n.a.	n.a.	n.a.	n.a.	n.a.	n.a.	n.a.
1943	3,295	3,197	3,182	11,802	5,836	7,803	3,118	427	1,887	1,700	7,667	49,914
1944	3,489	2,992	3,263	12,025	5,475	6,864	3,055	395	1,832	1,784	7,379	48,553
1945	3,199	2,879	3,402	13,207	5,314	8,874	3,050	417	2,123	1,790	7,775	52,030
1946	2,910	2,396	3,455	10,852	3,854	4,388	2,626	354	1,471	2,096	6,162	40,564
1947	2,885	2,130	3,785	10,564	4,277	3,975	2,668	413	1,427	2,213	6,163	40,500
1948	2,446	1,872	3,891	11,254	3,577	4,305	2,714	343	1,361	2,197	6,228	40,188
1949	2,314	1,671	4,063	12,034	3,574	3,950	2,835	349	1,413	2,063	6,274	40,540

Table 55—Continued

Groups of Causes

	I	II	III	IV	V	VI	VII	VIII	IX	X	XI	Total
1950	2,183	863	4,330	12,534	2,972	2,565	2,381	319	1,681	2,092	7,270	39,190
1951	2,172	968	4,533	12,992	3,404	3,482	2,555	329	1,793	2,112	6,599	40,939
1952	1,502	806	4,830	12,464	2,278	2,907	2,357	287	1,703	2,114	5,964	37,212
1953	1,128	755	5,003	12,953	2,452	2,762	2,213	260	1,625	1,922	6,104	37,177

Source: Cuban vital statistics.

I=respiratory tuberculosis; II=other infectious and parasitic diseases; III=malignant and benign tumors; IV=cardiovascular diseases; V=influenza, pneumonia, and bronchitis; VI=diarrhea, gastritis, and enteritis; VII=certain degenerative diseases; VIII=complications of pregnancy; IX=certain diseases of infancy; X=accidents and violence; XI=all other and unknown causes.

n.a. means data not available.

Table 56
Per Capita Consumption of Rice, Canned and Dry Milk,
and Insecticides, Cuba
(In Kilograms)

Year	Rice	Canned and Dry Milk	Insecticides
1902	43.3	1.97	
1903	36.9	1.84	
1904	47.4	2.32	
1905	50.5	3.18	
1906	44.1	3.87	
1907	57.6	4.65	
1908	47.4	3.89	
1909	50.7	4.08	
1910	52.2	5.68	
1911	51.6	6.06	
1912	50.4	5.66	
1913	52.2	6.14	
1914	45.3	5.97	
1915	55.3	6.12	
1916	62.0	5.99	
1917	52.8	6.02	
1918	61.3	6.33	
1919	49.8	6.31	
1920	71.9	7.74	
1921	37.5	6.20	
1922	55.2	5.81	
1923	61.6	6.43	
1924	60.2	6.40	
1925	55.9	6.24	
1926	61.5	6.26	
1927	54.8	6.36	
1928	n.a.	n.a.	
1929	n.a.	n.a.	
1930	53.2	4.57	0.02
1931	45.6	1.89	0.04
1932	40.1	1.28	0.02
1933	35.4	0.56	0.01
1934	44.4	0.29	0.03
1935	57.0	0.34	0.03
1936	50.9	0.52	0.04
1937	55.2	0.44	0.07
1938	46.0	0.57	0.05

Table 56—*Continued*

Year	Rice	Canned and Dry Milk	Insecticides
1939	48.6	0.09	0.07
1940	46.5	0.04	0.05
1941	40.5	5.31	0.10
1942	35.2	3.93	0.04
1943	43.9	3.45	0.08
1944	45.6	2.99	0.10
1945	42.7	2.47	0.24
1946	35.4	5.22	0.14
1947	35.0	2.30	0.15
1948	52.3	5.48	0.28
1949	57.8	7.08	0.18
1950	63.1	6.56	0.28
1951	64.1	6.82	0.30
1952	52.2	6.94	0.42
1953	60.6	6.35	0.31

Sources: *Comercio Exterior* and tables in Cuban Economic Research Project, *A Study on Cuba* (Coral Gables, Fla.: University of Miami, 1965).

Note: The series on canned and dry milk is misleading during the 1930s, since it does not take into account national production. Up to 1940, the figures refer only to imports. After that time imports and national production are considered.

n.a. means data not available.

Notes

Chapter 1. Introduction

1. Ansley J. Coale, "The History of the Human Population," *Scientific American* 231, no. 3 (September 1974):43.

2. John D. Durand, "Historical Estimates of World Population: An Evaluation," *Population and Development Review* 3, no. 3 (September 1977):259.

3. United Nations, *World Population Trends and Prospects by Country, 1950-2000: Summary Report of the 1978 Assessment*, ST/ESA/SER.R/33 (New York, 1979); and International Bank for Reconstruction and Development, *World Development Report, 1979* (Washington, D.C., August 1979).

4. France and Germany are notorious exceptions, since in these two countries declines in mortality and fertility began almost simultaneously (Ansley J. Coale, "The Demographic Transition," in *The Population Debate* [New York: United Nations, 1975], 1:350-351).

5. See George J. Stolnitz, "The Demographic Transition: From High to Low Birth Rates and Death Rates," in *Population: The Vital Revolution*, ed. Ronald Freedman (Garden City, N.Y.: Anchor Books, 1964), pp. 30-46, for transition theory with a focus on mortality; and Coale, "The Demographic Transition," for transition theory with a focus on fertility.

6. Abdel R. Omran, "The Epidemiologic Transition," *Milbank Memorial Fund Quarterly* 49, no. 4, pt. 1:509-538.

7. R. H. Gray, "The Decline of Mortality in Ceylon and the Demographic Effects of Malaria Control," *Population Studies* 28, no. 2 (July 1974):205-229; Peter Newman, *Malaria Eradication and Population Growth with Special Reference to Ceylon and British Guiana*, Bureau of Public Health Economics, Research Series no. 10 (University of Michigan School of Public Health, 1965).

8. These developments are reviewed in United Nations, Department of Social Affairs, *The Determinants and Consequences of Population Trends*, 2 vols. (New

York, 1973), 1:142-146.

9. Thomas McKeown, *The Modern Rise of Population* (London: Edward Arnold, 1976), p. 108.

10. P. E. Razzell, "'An Interpretation of the Modern Rise of Population in Europe'—A Critique," *Population Studies* 28, no. 1 (March 1974):5-17.

11. United Nations, *Determinants and Consequences*, 1:149-150.

12. See Thomas McKeown and R. G. Record, "Reasons for the Decline of Mortality in England and Wales during the Nineteenth Century," *Population Studies* 16, no. 2 (November 1962):94-122; Thomas McKeown, R. G. Record, and R. G. Brown, "An Interpretation of the Modern Rise of Population in Europe," *Population Studies* 26, no. 3 (November 1972):345-382; Thomas McKeown, R. G. Record, and R. D. Turner, "An Interpretation of the Decline of Mortality in England and Wales during the Twentieth Century," *Population Studies* 29, no. 3 (November 1975):391-422; and McKeown, *The Modern Rise of Population*.

13. Jay R. Mandle, "The Decline in Mortality in British Guiana, 1911-1960," *Demography* 7, no. 3 (August 1970):301-315.

14. Eduardo E. Arriaga and Kingsley Davis, "The Pattern of Mortality Change in Latin America," *Demography* 6, no. 3 (August 1969):223-242.

15. Samuel H. Preston, "The Changing Relation between Mortality and Level of Economic Development," *Population Studies* 29, no. 2 (July 1975):231-248.

16. United Nations, *Determinants and Consequences*, 1:118.

17. Samuel H. Preston and Verne E. Nelson, "Structure and Change in Causes of Death: An International Summary," *Population Studies* 28, no. 1 (March 1974):19-51.

Chapter 2. The Secular Trend of Mortality in Cuba

1. The number of deaths per one thousand population in a given year.

2. A life table is a statistical model that combines the mortality experience of different age-groups in a population. The resultant values serve to measure the probability of death, survivorship, and life expectancy. The table's best-known summary measure, life expectancy at birth, may be interpreted as the average number of years a person born under the mortality conditions prevalent at the time of his birth may be expected to live.

3. A classic description of these techniques is provided in United Nations, Department of Social Affairs, *Methods of Estimating Basic Demographic Measures from Incomplete Data*, ST/SOA/Series A/42 (New York, 1967).

4. Guy Bourdé, "Fuentes y métodos de la historia demográfica en Cuba (Siglo XVIII y XIX)," *Revista de la Biblioteca Nacional José Martí* 16, no. 1 (December 1975):21-68.

5. Hugh Thomas, *Cuba: The Pursuit of Freedom*, (New York: Harper & Row, 1971), p. 423. A more detailed discussion of living conditions in Cuba during the war period is provided in Chapter 3, pp. 27-28.

6. A census was not actually taken in 1901. However, since detailed mortality data first become available in that year, it was decided to project the population of

Havana enumerated in 1899 up to 1901 utilizing the estimated intercensal rate of growth and assuming the continuation of a similar age structure.

7. Of the 174,221 migrants recorded entering Cuba in 1920, 163,949, or 94.1 percent, were males.

8. Rodolfo Mezquita, *Cuba: Estimación de la mortalidad por sexo. Tabla de vida para los períodos 1919-31 y 1931-43*, series c, no. 121 (Santiago, Chile: Centro Latinoamericano de Demografía, March 1970); and Fernando González Q. and Jorge Debasa, *Cuba: Evaluación y ajuste del censo de 1953 y las estadísticas de nacimientos y defunciones entre 1943 y 1958. Tabla de mortalidad por sexo, 1952-54*, series C, no. 124 (Santiago, Chile: Centro Latinoamericano de Demografía, 1970).

9. I projected the enumerated population in 1907 to 1909 in order to obtain two ten-year intervals needed for the application of the estimating technique that was used. The results of these life tables are in basic agreement with other life tables estimated for roughly the same dates by the Centro de Estudios Demográficos of the University of Havana and based on the interpolation of the values estimated by Mezquita, *Cuba: Estimación de la mortalidad*, and González Q. and Debasa, *Cuba: Evaluación y ajuste del censo*, and the derivation of other life tables. Elio Velázquez and Lázaro Toirao, *Cuba: Tablas de mortalidad estimadas por sexo, para los años calendarios terminados en cero y cinco durante el período 1900-1950*, Estudios Demográficos, series 1, no. 3 (Havana: Centro de Estudios Demográficos, Instituto de Economía, University of Havana, July 1975) provides the life-table estimates derived from those estimated by Mezquita and González Q. and Debasa.

10. Junta Central de Planificación (JUCEPLAN), *La esperanza o expectativa de vida*, Havana: JUCEPLAN, 1974.

11 Centro Latinoamericano de Demografía (San José), and Dirección de Demografía, Comité Estatal de Estadísticas (Cuba), "Proyección de la población cubana 1950-2000, nivel nacional: Metodología y resultados" (Havana, August 1978), p. 35.

12. The Uruguayan experience probably approximates that of Argentina, but no dependable series of life expectancy estimates is available. Jamaica, Barbados, and other Caribbean countries have mortality experiences comparable in some respects to Cuba's.

13. An obvious exception to this generalization is Puerto Rico, since it has a life expectancy even higher than that reached by the United States and other developed countries. However, because of its peculiar political and economic status, it is inappropriate to make comparisons between the island and the rest of Latin America. For the reader's information, the trend in life expectancy for both sexes combined for Puerto Rico is presented below:

Year	Life Expectancy	Year	Life Expectancy
1903	30.4	1949-51	60.9
1909-11	38.2	1959-61	69.4
1919-21	38.5	1969-71	71.9
1929-31	40.6	1974-76	73.2
1939-41	46.0		

Source: José L. Vásquez Calzada, *La población de Puerto Rico y su trayectoria histórica* (San Juan: Centro Multidisciplinario de Estudios Poblacionales, 1978), p. 232.

Chapter 3. The Premodern Period and the Initial Mortality Decline

1. For a description of the economic events at the time, see, for example, Hugh Thomas, *Cuba: The Pursuit of Freedom*, (New York: Harper & Row, 1971), pp. 109-135.

2. Estimates vary, but scholars believe that at least 420,000 slaves were imported to Cuba between 1800 and 1865. Over 120,000 indentured laborers found their way into the country between 1847 and 1873 (ibid., pp. 1532-1533, 1541.) The population doubled approximately every thirty years, although mortality was very high: from 272,000 in 1792, to slightly over 700,000 in 1827, to nearly 1,400,000 in 1861.

3. So notoriously unhealthy were the conditions in nineteenth-century Cuba, that historian Willis Fletcher Johnson noted that Cuba was a place that insurance companies prohibited their policyholders to visit (*The History of Cuba*, 5 vols. [New York: B. F. Buck & Co., 1920], 4:177).

4. See, for example, Richard Gallagher, *Diseases that Plague Modern Man*, (Dobbs Ferry, N. Y.: Oceana Publications, 1969), pp. 21-25.

5. Jorge Le-Roy y Cassá, *Estudios sobre la mortalidad de la Habana durante el siglo XIX y los comienzos del actual*, (Havana: Imprenta Lloredo, 1913).

6. Ibid., pp. 10-14.

7. Ross Danielson discusses health standards in Havana during the nineteenth century in *Cuban Medicine* (New Brunswick, N. J.: Transaction Books, 1979), pp. 85-89.

8. Yellow fever was regarded as particularly lethal to the nonimmune foreign born. In December 1900, for instance, of the 119 cases of yellow fever in Havana, 57, or almost 50 percent, were individuals who had been in the country less than three years. Over half of the 57 cases (31 cases) had been in the country less than three months. Twenty of the 119 cases died; of those, 19 were Spanish and one was American (*Revista de Medicina y Cirugía de la Habana* 6, no. 2 [25 January 1901]:39-40).

9. Thomas, *Cuba: The Pursuit of Freedom*, p. 175.

10. Kenneth F. Kiple, *Blacks in Colonial Cuba, 1774-1899* (Gainesville: University Presses of Florida, 1976), pp. 54-55. Kiple's discussion indicates how uncertain estimates of slave mortality were, however.

11. Franklin W. Knight, *Slave Society in Cuba during the Nineteenth Century* (Madison: University of Wisconsin Press, 1970), p. 82.

12. That smallpox, by then a fully controllable disease, took so many lives indicates how negligent the Spanish colonial authorities were. In 1804, just eight years after Jenner's vaccination experiment, the technique began to be used in Cuba. From February 1804 to November 1835, 210,579 persons were vaccinated in Havana and a total of 311,342 persons in the whole country (Emilio Roig de Leuchsenring, "En el centenario de Tomás Romay," *Sanidad y Beneficencia Municipal* 9, no. 1 [January-March 1949]:20-24). It is interesting that the first recorded flare-up of smallpox during the nineteenth century occurred in 1870, a war year. More interesting still, the major attacks took place during the peacetime years,

1878 to 1894 (the so-called Ten Years War ended in 1878), particularly in 1878, 1881, and 1887. One wonders if the gradual phasing out of slavery between 1880 and 1886 had something to do with the spread of smallpox, since, perhaps, the better-informed slave owners decided not to continue vaccinating the property that they were about to lose. Kiple observes that one of the causes of the drastic decline in the slave population between 1861 and 1887 may have been the "desperate slave owners reacting to the impending end of slavery by overworking their slaves" (Kiple, *Blacks in Colonial Cuba*, p. 81).

13. Infants appear to be particularly susceptible to diphtheria. See Abram S. Benenson, ed., *Control of Communicable Diseases in Man*, 11th ed., (Washington, D.C.: American Public Health Association, 1970), pp. 77-82.

14. Thomas, *Cuba: The Pursuit of Freedom*, pp. 334, 1562-1563.

15. Philip S. Foner, *The Spanish-Cuban-American War and the Birth of American Imperialism* (New York: Monthly Review Press, 1972), 2:379. Foner provides one of the most vivid descriptions of the extent of destruction that the war brought to Cuba and its people. See especially pp. 379-387.

16. Ibid., p. 381.

17. The (probably) very reliable figures quoted by Thomas regarding the military losses of the Spanish and American armies indicate how inhospitable conditions were in Cuba during the war period and immediately after the hostilities ceased. The Spanish army reported having lost 62,853 between 1895 and 1898. Of these, 53,440, or 85 percent, died of yellow fever or other diseases, while only about 15 percent were killed in action or died of wounds received in combat. The American forces lost 5,509 soldiers to disease, out of a total of 6,212 war deaths, or 88.7 percent, from March 1898 to June 1899 (Thomas, *Cuba: The Pursuit of Freedom*, pp. 405, 414.

18. W. C. Gorgas, "Office of Chief Sanitary Officer for Havana, Report to the Adjutant General, May 8, 1900," *Civil Report of Brigadier Leonard Wood, Military Governor of Cuba, 1901*, 9 vols. (Washington, D.C.: Government Printing Office, 1902), 4:7.

19. After the National Center for Vaccination was established in 1901, it was reported that between September 1 of that year and January 31 of 1902, 265,672 vaccinations and revaccinations were made throughout the country (Vicente de la Guardia, "Algunas consideraciones acerca del servicio de la vacuna antivariolosa en Cuba," *Sanidad y Beneficencia* vol. 19, no. 2 [February 1918]:124. Among other sources that provide indications of the nationwide vaccination program, see P. G. Betancourt, "Report of the Civil Government of the Province of Matanzas," and Guillermo Dolz, "Report Presented by the Civil Governor of Pinar del Río, of the Present Condition of the Province and of the Public Service and Administrative Work Performed in the Same during the Fiscal Year of 1899-1900," both in *Civil Report of Brigadier Leonard Wood, Military Governor of Cuba, 1901* 3:3-21 and 5-29 (page numbers are not consecutive). Secondary sources, such as Johnson, *The History of Cuba*; Thomas, *Cuba: The Pursuit of Freedom*; Foner, *The Spanish-Cuban-American War*; and many others also provide evidence of the island-wide

sanitary programs.

20. W. C. Gorgas, "Office of Chief Sanitary Officer of Havana, Report to the Adjutant General, February 5, 1901," *Civil Report of Brigadier Leonard Wood, Military Governor of Cuba, 1901* 4:9-10. A better idea of the magnitude of the cleaning effort may be conveyed by indicating that the city of Havana had at the time a total of 26,701 dwellings.

21. Gorgas, "May 8, 1900," 4:4-8; idem, "February 5, 1901," 4:3-15; and V. Havard, "Sanitation and Yellow Fever in Havana, February 8, 1901," *Civil Report of Brigadier Leonard Wood, Military Governor of Cuba, 1901*, 4:3-15.

22. The classic experimental conditions under which the links between yellow fever, mosquitoes, and man were established have been frequently described. For a detailed exposition of how the Yellow Fever Commission, under the direction of Walter Reed, proceeded in its task, see Johnson, *The History of Cuba*, pp. 171-177. For a briefer but more accessible exposition, see George Rosen, *A History of Public Health* (New York: MD Publications, 1958), pp. 325-326. Earlier cleaning campaigns had been primarily geared to the elimination of yellow fever, which at the time was believed to be produced by, or to be associated with, filth. After verifying early in February 1901 that mosquitoes, and not filth, were responsible for the transmission of yellow fever, efforts and available resources were redirected toward fighting the actual sources of the disease. The benefits of the clean-up campaign in reducing other infectious diseases are obvious.

23. Gordon Harrison, *Mosquitoes, Malaria and Man: A History of the Hostilities since 1880* (New York: E. P. Dutton, 1978), p. 162.

24. Similar improvements may have been instituted simultaneously in Puerto Rico and the Philippines, but they do not seem to be as well documented. In reference to Puerto Rico, Kingsley Davis notes that "since 1900 great effort has been made to reduce the death rate." However, the data that he presents seem to indicate that the decline had started much earlier, in the late 1800s. In view of the Cuban evidence, the validity of the data showing an earlier mortality decline in Puerto Rico should be suspected (Kingsley Davis, "Puerto Rico: A Crowded Island," *Annals of the American Academy of Political and Social Sciences* 285 [January 1953]:116-122). A later example, very well known but, as far as I know, not quantified, occurred in Panama during the construction of the canal early in the present century. Another case, better documented than that for Cuba, occurred in Taiwan a few years after Cuban sanitary reform. The similarities between the sanitary reforms instituted in Taiwan by the Japanese and those in Cuba by the Americans are considerable. It appears that the tempo of the decline was faster in Cuba than in Taiwan (George W. Barclay, *Colonial Development and Population in Taiwan* [1954; reprint ed., Port Washington, N. Y.: Kennikat Press, 1972], pp. 133-172).

25. The extent to which sanitation expenditures alone increased during this period is made clear by what a Havana newspaper stated regarding the way in which custom receipts (from which the Cuban budgets primarily originated) were allocated. It was observed that from July to December 1899, in the city of Havana exclusively, 1,688,442 pesos had been spent for sanitary purposes. By contrast, during the years

when the country had been a Spanish colony, no more than 200,000 pesos were normally assigned to sanitation (*Diario de la Marina*, 24 May 1900, p. 2). Obviously, the conditions found in the country after the end of the war contributed to the large differential. During the whole period of the military occupation, July 18, 1898 to May 19, 1902, 20,358,607 pesos, or over 36 percent of total government expenditures, went to sanitation or sanitation-related areas (quarantine, 694,024 pesos; 5,833,607 for public works; 4,124,986 for hospitals and rest homes; and 9,706,258 pesos for sanitation). These figures are given in Cuban Economic Research Project, *A Study on Cuba* (Coral Gables, Fla.: University of Miami Press, 1965), p. 166.

26. Improvement in nutrition may have contributed to some decline in tuberculosis mortality. However, it is questionable whether this would have been the case in the absence of the war conditions.

Chapter 4. The Context of the Mortality Decline in the First Half of the Twentieth Century

1. This view is substantiated by many direct references in the literature, as well as by the many documents concerning public health that were published in English in Cuba, obviously aimed at the American audience. A discussion of some of these issues may be found in David A. Lockmiller, *Magoon in Cuba: A History of the Second Intervention, 1906-1909* (Chapel Hill: University of North Carolina Press, 1938), pp. 22-24, 112-119.

2. Archibald R. M. Ritter, *The Economic Development of Revolutionary Cuba: Strategy and Performance* (New York: Praeger Publishers, 1975), pp. 16-18.

3. For a general discussion of these events by a Cuban medical historian, see César Rodríguez y Exposito, *La primera secretaría de sanidad del mundo se creó en Cuba*, Cuadernos de Historia de Salud Pública, no. 25 (Havana, 1964). The Cuban literature of the time discusses in detail why these reforms were instituted.

4. Cuban Economic Research Project, *A Study on Cuba* (Coral Gables, Fla.: University of Miami Press, 1965), pp. 280, 403, and 616.

5. International Bank for Reconstruction and Development (World Bank), *Report on Cuba* (Baltimore, Md.: Johns Hopkins University Press, 1951), p. 45. The large fluctuations in percentage of total national income originating in the milling and marketing of this commodity from year to year were produced by an increase in production from 3.4 million tons of sugar in 1945 to 5.6 million tons in 1949.

6. We can gain an idea of the growth of the economy during these years by realizing that "the value of United States investments in Cuba, which in 1911 had amounted to 205 million dollars, attained a figure of 1,140 million dollars in the year 1927" (Cuban Economic Research Project, *A Study on Cuba*, p. 293). The greater part of these investments went into the sugar industry. Investments from other countries, mainly England and Canada, were also substantial, but far less than those from the United States. Foreign ownership of national wealth increased significantly during the early 1920s, when local banks failed, causing the bankruptcy of numerous

national firms (Ritter, *Economic Development*, p. 17).

7. Henry Christopher Wallich, *Monetary Problems of an Export Economy: The Cuban Experience, 1914-1917* (Cambridge, Mass.: Harvard University Press, 1950), p. 11.

8. International Bank for Reconstruction and Development, *Report on Cuba*, pp. 57-58.

9. These views are only briefly summarized here, since they are well known and since a detailed discussion is well beyond the scope of this study. See, for comprehensive discussions of the development of the Cuban economy, James O'Connor, *The Origins of Socialism in Cuba* (Ithaca, N. Y.: Cornell University Press, 1970); Julio Le Riverend Brusone, *Economic History of Cuba* (Havana: Ensayo Book Institute, 1967); and Comisión Económica para América Latina (CEPAL), *Cuba: Estilo de desarrollo y políticas sociales* (Mexico City: Siglo Veintiuno, 1980).

10. Julián Alienes y Urosa, *Características fundamentales de la economía cubana* (Havana: Banco Nacional de Cuba, 1950), p. 2.

11. International Bank for Reconstruction and Development, *Report on Cuba*, p. 1047.

12. Ibid., p. 40.

13. However, the World Bank study noted that "the general impression of members of the Mission, from observations in travels all over Cuba, is that living levels of the farmers, agricultural laborers, industrial workers, storekeepers, and others, are higher all along the line than for corresponding groups in other tropical countries and in nearly all other Latin American countries. This does not mean that there is no dire poverty in Cuba, but simply that in comparative terms Cubans are better off, on the average, than the people of these other areas" (International Bank for Reconstruction and Development, *Report on Cuba*, pp. 39-40). Note, however, that this assessment was made at a fairly prosperous time (around 1950).

14. The case can be made that a large percentage of dwellings receiving their water supplies from wells may signify a relative improvement, on the assumption that wells may supply a steady and, if treated, safe supply of water. However, evidence to be discussed later makes such an assumption questionable.

15. These percentages are described as "no less than" because there is a residual category where "other combinations," without further elaboration, are given.

16. República de Cuba, *Censo de 1953*, pp. xxxi, 211, and 213. Lowry Nelson, in his classic study of conditions in rural Cuba, estimated that a typical Cuban rural dwelling could be built for about two hundred dollars, hardly an amount suggestive of a comfortable or sanitary house (*Rural Cuba* [1950; reprint ed., New York: Octagon Books, 1970], p. 204).

17. See José Antonio López del Valle, *The Development of Sanitation and Charities in Cuba during the Last Sixteen Years (1899-1914)* (Havana:Moderna Poesía, 1914).

18. Lockmiller, *Magoon in Cuba*, pp. 117-121.

19. República de Cuba, *Census 1919*, p. 193.

20. República de Cuba, *Censo de 1943*, pp. 360-362.

21. Ibid., pp. 354-361.

22. International Bank for Reconstruction and Development, *Report on Cuba*, p. 328. Even in the City of Havana the water supply was impure. Most upper- and middle-income groups obtained their drinking water from private suppliers who made home deliveries of spring water. Theirs was a thriving business.

23. The reversal in the trend of increasing percentages of the total population in the metropolitan area of Havana, in 1919, may have resulted from heavy immigration or the expansion of the sugar industry into previously sparsely settled parts of the country about that time.

24. Wyatt MacGaffey and Clifford R. Barnett, *Cuba, Its People, Its Society, Its Culture* (1962; reprint ed., Westport, Conn.: Greenwood Press, 1974), p. 164.

25. Ibid., pp. 164-165. The same observation recurs in other literature on Cuba. Nelson noted the tendency in the Cuban diet to rely on starchy food (*Rural Cuba*, p. 208); and the World Bank observed that "even wealthy Cubans eat too much of the wrong kind" (International Bank for Reconstruction and Development, *Report on Cuba*, p. 446.)

26. Norman Jolliffe, Robert S. Goodhart, Morton Archer, Hady López, and Flavio Galbán Díaz, "Nutrition Status Survey of the Sixth Grade School Population of Cuba," *Journal of Nutrition*, 64, no. 3 (March 1958):355-398.

27. Ibid., pp. 365, 394.

28. International Bank for Reconstruction and Development, *Report on Cuba*, pp. 446-447.

29. Agrupación Católica Universitaria, "Encuesta de trabajadores rurales, 1956-57," *Economía y Desarrollo*, no. 12 (July-August 1972), pp. 188-213.

30. The data on rice imports were obtained from the yearly volumes of República de Cuba, *Comercio Exterior*, Havana. This yearly series runs from 1902 to 1958. A two-year gap in the series (1928 and 1929) was filled by assuming that the trends shown for earlier and later years prevailed during those years. The data on national production were taken from the figures given in Cuban Economic Research Project, *A Study on Cuba*.

31. This conclusion has been reached by inspecting the census returns for local areas (not shown in the table), and other evidence discussed later.

32. Foreign Policy Association, *Problems of the New Cuba* (New York: J. J. Little & Ives Co., 1935), p. 118.

33. Ross Danielson, *Cuban Medicine*, (New Brunswick, N.J.: Transaction Books, 1979), pp. 110-113, shows figures that indicate that in 1934 there were in Cuba thirty-six national and municipal hospitals, of which twenty-six were located outside of the Province of Havana.

34. Manuel F. Alonso, "La beneficencia en Cuba: Casas de salud," *Sanidad y Beneficencia* 12, no. 2 (August 1914):178-209; and 12, no. 4 (October 1914):471-475.

35. R. G. Leland, "The Practice of Medicine in Cuba," *American Medical Association Bulletin* (June 1933), p. 92. This source notes that the membership of the mutualist associations declined significantly, by as much as 70 percent in some of

the clinics, during years of economic crisis.

36. Ibid., p. 92. These associations extended even to Key West and Tampa, Florida, where many Cubans and Spanish-born residents of Cuba went when labor problems in Cuba led to the relocation of many cigar factories. Some of them have survived. Clinics along the same organizational lines have been established in the Miami, Florida, area and are very active today among the large Cuban population that left Cuba after the 1959 revolution. In Cuba they have disappeared, since all medical services are now under official control.

37. Danielson suggests that the mutualist associations may have been as important, if not more important, than the government sector in providing health services to the population, at least in Havana and other large urban centers (*Cuban Medicine*).

38. These statistics appear in the yearly volumes of República de Cuba, *Comercio Exterior*, mentioned in note 30.

Chapter 5. The Mortality Decline in Havana, 1901-1953

1. The estimated infant mortality rates for all years apear to be too low, particularly in 1907, 1919, and 1931. The infant mortality rates for these three years were computed after adjusting for underenumeration of young children. However, the adjustments seem to overcompensate for the noted underenumeration. Despite these biases, the life expectancy trends and the trends of cause-specific mortality, computed with these rates, are only slightly disturbed, and therefore do not affect the major conclusions of the study. For further details, see the Statistical Appendix, especially table 53, in which cause-specific death rates computed with the unadjusted population data are shown.

2. Thomas McKeown, R. G. Record, and R. D. Turner, "An Interpretation of the Decline of Mortality in England and Wales during the Twentieth Century," *Population Studies* 29, no. 3(November 1975):393.

3. This technique has been used by McKeown, Record, and Turner. It consists of estimating the number of lives that would have been saved after standardizing by age and sex to the original population. The standard population used was the one for the earlier period, either 1901 or 1907. It should be noted that choosing any other standard population for these calculations may produce somewhat different results. Much of the analysis that follows regarding changes by age and cause during the mortality transition in Havana is based, methodologically, on ibid.

4. Since the Cuban statistics on death by cause during the 1901-1953 period were coded according to the first six revisions of the International List of Causes of Death, I had to group the data in order to make the series comparable and to reduce the number of categories to a manageable size. I used the grouping scheme devised by Samuel H. Preston, Nathan Keyfitz, and Robert Schoen, with some minor adjustments of my own (*Causes of Death: Life Tables for National Populations* [New York: Seminar Press, 1972]).

5. Of the more specific causes, eleven are included in the major group "other infectious and parasitic diseases," one in the group "certain degenerative diseases,"

and two in the residual group "all others and unknown."

6. I obtained the estimated percentage declines by using the age-sex or age-standardized cause-specific death rates.

7. Samuel H. Preston and Verne E. Nelson, "Structure and Change in Causes of Death: An International Summary," *Population Studies* 28, no. 1 (March 1974):29-30.

8. I had to use the data for 1907, since the age groupings by cause of death available for 1901 were very different from those published in 1953. Even when the 1907 data are used, the comparison is only approximate, since the age groups at the two dates do not match exactly. Some age groups are similar, but others overlap. The biases should not be significant, since the overlaps are in narrow age ranges in which the force of mortality varies only slightly. The age groups available for 1907 are as follows, with those for 1953 in parentheses: under one (under one); one to four (one to four); five to fourteen (five to fourteen); fifteen to twenty-nine (fifteen to twenty-four); thirty to forty-four (twenty-five to forty-four); forty-five to fifty-nine (forty-five to sixty-four); sixty to seventy-four (sixty-five to seventy-four); and seventy-five and over (seventy-five and over). In the text and the table, I refer to the age groups for 1907.

9. Samuel H. Preston, *Mortality Patterns in National Populations* (New York: Academic Press, 1976), pp. 89-102.

10. Hugo Behm, "Recent Mortality Trends in Chile," Vital and Health Statistics, Analytical Studies, series 3, no. 2 (Washington, D.C.: National Center for Health Statistics, April 1964).

Chapter 6. The Decline of Mortality from Specific Causes

1. Anthony M. Lowell, Lydia B. Edwards, and Carrol E. Palmer, *Tuberculosis*, Vital and Health Statistics Monographs, American Public Health Association, (Cambridge, Mass.: Harvard University Press, 1969); Thomas McKeown and R. G. Record, "Reasons for the Decline of Mortality in England and Wales during the Nineteenth Century," *Population Studies* 16, no. 2 (November 1962):94-122; Thomas McKeown, R. G. Record, and R. D. Turner, "An Interpretation of the Decline of Mortality in England and Wales during the Twentieth Century," *Population Studies* 29, no. 3 (November 1975):391-422; Elizabeth Newell, "The Sources of Mortality Changes in Italy since Unification," (Ph.D. diss., University of Pennsylvania, 1972).

2. José Antonio López del Valle, *The Development of Sanitation and Charities in Cuba during the Last Sixteen Years (1899-1914)* (Havana: Moderna Poesía, 1914).

3. See Nicolás Gómez de Rosas, "Plan de abastecimiento de leche," *Sanidad y Beneficencia* 12, no. 6 (December 1914):663-695, for a good example.

4. "Mensaje presidencial," *Sanidad y Beneficencia* 33, nos. 1-12 (January-December 1928):333.

5. Ibid., p. 338.

6. "El Consejo Nacional de Tuberculosis," in *El consejo corporativo de*

educación, sanidad y beneficencia y sus instituciones filiales. Resumen de lo que son y lo que hacen, ed. Arístides Sosa de Quesada (Havana: Instituto Cívico-Militar, 1937), pp. 115-140.

7. República de Cuba, *Censo de 1943* (Havana, 1945), pp. 525-530.

8. It may be argued that the rates of nonrespiratory tuberculosis did decline significantly between 1901 (or 1907) and 1919. The difference between the rates for 1901 and 1919 amounts to close to 30 percent, and the difference is even larger between 1907 and 1919. Such findings are consistent with the evidence on the implementation of measures designed to minimize the impact of direct contagion through contaminated milk. However, since nonrespiratory tuberculosis can be acquired from human as well as bovine sources, and since the time interval between the implementation of measures against bovine forms of the disease and the actual decline in mortality rates is fairly short, this interpretation can only be held as tentative.

9. I have adopted this approach, instead of the calculation of cause-specific death rates from the statistics for all Cuba and non-Havana Cuba, as a way of minimizing the distortion of comparisons due to underregistration of deaths outside Havana. Its validity depends on the assumption that the relative degrees of underregistration of deaths from various causes did not change significantly over time. For example, if tuberculosis deaths were more underregistered than deaths from other causes on the average, but the relative degree of underregistration of tuberculosis deaths in comparison with others was approximately the same at different dates, then the comparison of trends over time in the percentages of deaths attributed to tuberculosis in Havana and in non-Havana Cuba should indicate whether or not the trends of tuberculosis mortality rates outside the capital city were approximately parallel with the trends in Havana. The percentages of deaths attributed to various causes have been calculated according to the all-inclusive grouping of causes of deaths formulated by Samuel H. Preston, Nathan Keyfitz, and Robert Schoen in *Causes of Death: Life Tables for National Populations* (New York: Seminar Press, 1972). Approaches similar to mine have been used on other occasions, but, as far as I know, never exactly this way and never covering such a long time interval. See, for example, Jean Bourgeois-Pichet and Chia-Lin Pan, "Trends and Determinants of Mortality in Underdeveloped Areas," in *Trends and Differentials in Mortality* (New York: Milbank Memorial Fund, 1956), pp. 11-25.

10. This is consistent with the city's heavy population concentration in the mid-range of the age structure, where tuberculosis mortality is highest, and with the location of tuberculosis hospitals in Havana, which results in the recording of deaths of nonresidents there. Another reason for the higher percentages of tuberculosis mortality in the city may be greater rates of contagion in a large city with high population density.

11. The questionable quality of the demographic data constantly raises questions of interpretation. It is possible that the apparent reversal in the trend of age-sex-standardized tuberculosis mortality rates for Havana is a statistical artifact, since the tuberculosis survey carried out during the late 1930s led to the identification of many

new cases of tuberculosis. This may have resulted in the treatment of many of the afflicted in the hospital facilities of the capital, where any deaths would have been registered on a de facto basis. We can use a similar argument to explain the increases in the percentages of deaths attributed to tuberculosis. In spite of these confounding factors, my feeling is that the main interpretations that I have reached concerning the trends of tuberculosis mortality are not substantially altered.

12. Thomas McKeown, R. G. Record, and R. D. Turner, "An Interpretation of the Decline of Mortality in England and Wales during the Twentieth Century," *Population Studies* 29, no. 3 (November 1975):391-422.

13. Henry P. Carr, Rolla B. Hill, Joaquín Fernández Meléndez, Alberto Ros, and Arístides Fernández Meléndez, *Reconocimiento de paludismo en Cuba* (Havana: Instituto Finlay, 1943). A series of articles published in the *American Journal of Tropical Medicine* between 1940 and 1942 provides the results of the study in English. Although this survey was concerned with malaria morbidity, its results are relevant to the present study.

14. The spleen rate in Cuba was found to range in the different provinces from 8 to 16 percent. Less than half of one percent of the total number of children whose blood was examined were found to have parasites. In Ceylon (present-day Sri Lanka), the rates were generally much higher, reaching in some regions 67 percent. In Ceylon, the parasite rates ranged from 1.9 to 11.5 percent. The spleen rate was found to be as high as 74 percent in some districts of British Guiana (now Guyana) (R. H. Gray, "The Decline of Mortality in Ceylon and the Demographic Effects of Malaria Control," *Population Studies* 28, no. 2 [July 1974]:210; and Peter Newman, *Malaria Eradication and Population Growth with Special Reference to Ceylon and British Guiana*, Bureau of Public Health Economics, Research Series, no. 10 [Ann Arbor: University of Michigan, 1965], p. 135).

15. Carr et al., *Reconocimiento de paludismo*, pp. 73-74.

16. Abram S. Benenson, ed., *Control of Communicable Diseases in Man*, 11th ed. (Washington, D.C.: American Public Health Association, 1970), pp. 140-145.

17. This opinion was voiced by many writers on public health affairs in Cuba and appears to have been based on fact. As early as 1918 posters and pamphlets were distributed to the foreign laborers, printed in their own language, describing measures that could be taken to avoid malaria and informing the laborers that quinine could be obtained at no charge from the national sanitary authorities or from the large sugar mills that employed them (see, for example, "Anti-Malaria Campaign to English-Speaking Laborers," *Sanidad y Beneficencia* 19, no. 6 [June 1918]:531-533). In my opinion, excessive blame was placed on these laborers for the spread of malaria. To some extent, at least, the expansion of the sugar fields into more-distant areas may have contributed. Carr et al. found that in some of the last areas brought under cultivation, the conditions were conducive to endemic malaria. However, there is evidence that suggests that the immigrants brought other diseases with them.

18. Mainly for racial considerations, migrants from these areas were for years barred from entering Cuba (Asians were also barred). Since European migrants were

not prone to work in the sugar fields (with the exception of certain groups of temporary laborers), when the labor demand exceeded the supply, it was necessary to relax the immigration laws. These laws were first put on the Cuban books by the American occupation government. It has been said that their intention was to preserve the racial composition of the country, since the "whiter" it was, the more easily it could become an American state.

19. These were the standard measures instituted whenever malaria epidemics appeared. In all cases, and eventually by law, the private sector was brought into the sanitary plans, since it was expected to provide quinine, mosquito netting, and medical assistance, all free of charge, to the seasonal rural laborers. See, for example, Isidoro Agostini and Mario G. Lebredo, "Plan de campaña antipalúdica," *Sanidad y Beneficencia* 33, nos. 1-12 (January-December 1928):243-266.

20. McKeown, Record, and Turner, "Interpretation of the Decline," p. 412.

21. Benenson, *Control of Communicable Diseases*, p. 281.

22. McKeown, Record, and Turner, "Interpretation of the Decline," p. 414.

23. Benenson, *Control of Communicable Diseases*, pp. 145-146.

24. Two pieces of evidence support this interpretation. One is the rise in the population's literacy level during the first third of the century. The other is the frequent publication and free distribution by the sanitary authorities of pamphlets to educate the public in the ways of avoiding infectious diseases. Pamphlets dealing with scarlet fever, smallpox, typhoid fever, etc., were produced and distributed throughout the 1900-1953 period.

25. See Angel Argudín García, "La tos ferina en nuestro medio. Vacunación preventiva," *Revista de Sanidad y Beneficencia Municipal* (October-December 1941), pp. 103-108.

26. Carl C. Dauer, Robert F. Korns, and Leonard W. Schuman, *Infectious Diseases*, Vital and Health Statistics Monograph, American Public Health Association (Cambridge, Mass.: Harvard University Press, 1968), p. 25; and Newell, *Sources of Mortality Changes*, p. 112.

27. Benenson, *Control of Communicable Diseases*, pp. 220-221.

28. McKeown, Record, and Turner, "Interpretation of the Decline," p. 418.

29. Benenson, *Control of Communicable Diseases*, p. 222.

30. Ibid., p. 154.

31. Dauer, Korns, and Schuman, *Infectious Diseases*, p. 63.

32. Ibid., p. 60.

33. Benenson, *Control of Communicable Diseases*, p. 252.

34. The following figures are for Havana:

Year	All tetanus deaths	Neonatorum tetanus deaths
1900	191	125
1901	150	128
1902	97	68
1903	54	41
1904	52	33
1905	46	26
1906	45	25

Year	All tetanus deaths	Neonatorum tetanus deaths
1907	46	25
1908	43	18
1909	33	19
1910	22	9
1911	29	8
1912	27	12

The decline in the death rate from neonatorum tetanus was probably even more remarkable than the above figures show, since the absolute number of births probably increased phenomenally after the end of the war (Jorge Le-Roy y Cassá, "Desenvolvimiento de la sanidad en Cuba durante los últimos cincuenta años [1871-1920]," *Sanidad y Beneficencia* 26, nos. 1-12 [January-December 1921]:372).

35. A surviving pamphlet from this period is Junta Nacional de Sanidad y Beneficencia, *Higiene de la primera infancia: Instrucciones populares sobre la manera de cuidar a los niños* (Havana, 1905). Special attention was given in that booklet to the proper practices to follow in order to avoid neonatorum tetanus, referred to in Cuba as *el mal* (loosely translated as "the evil").

36. McKeown, Record, and Turner, "Interpretation of the Decline," p. 412.

37. Newell, *Sources of Mortality Changes*, p. 109.

38. See Andrés Garcia Rivera, "La organización sanitaria actual y reglas para su funcionamiento," *Sanidad y Beneficencia* 29, nos. 7-9 (July-September, 1924):356.

39. McKeown, Record, and Turner, "Interpretation of the Decline," pp. 418-419.

40. For a brief discussion of the social factors biasing the statistical records on syphilis mortality, see United Nations, *Foetal, Infant and Early Childhood Mortality*, vol. 1, *The Statistics* (New York, 1954), p. 48. For a more extensive discussion, emphasizing the problem associated with changes in medical knowledge and statistical approaches, see William J. Brown, James F. Donohue, Norman W. Axnick, Joseph H. Blount, Oscar G. Jones, and Neal H. Ewen, *Syphilis and Other Venereal Diseases*, Vital and Health Statistics Monograph, American Public Health Association (Cambridge, Mass.: Harvard University Press, 1970), pp. 17-57.

41. Rafael Calvo Fonseca, *El parasitismo intestinal en las zonas rurales de Cuba* (Havana: Instituto Finlay, 1953).

42. Rafael Calvo Fonseca, Raúl Cano Padrón, and Maria T. Calvo Miret, "Diez años de trabajos en la campaña contra el parasitismo intestinal," *Salubridad y Asistencia Social* 61, nos. 1-12 (January-December, 1958):13.

43. Benenson, *Control of Communicable Diseases*, p. 4.

44. Preston, Keyfitz, and Schoen, *Causes of Death*, p. 7.

45. Samuel H. Preston and Verne E. Nelson, "Structure and Change in Causes of Death: An International Summary," *Population Studies*, 28, no. 1 (March 1974):30.

46. Ibid., p. 30.

47. McKeown, Record, and Turner, "Interpretation of the Decline," p. 408.

48. Dauer, Korns, and Schuman, *Infectious Diseases*, pp. 170-171.

49. Ibid., p. 181.

50. McKeown, Record, and Turner, "Interpretation of the Decline," p. 410.

51. Ibid., pp. 415-416.

52. United Nations, Department of Social Affairs, *Foetal, Infant and Early Childhood Mortality*, 1:48.

53. This summary is based on discussions of gastroenteritis in Benenson, *Control of Communicable Diseases*, pp. 74-76; Pan American Health Organization, *Control of Gastrointestinal Diseases* (Washington, D.C., 1964); McKeown, Record, and Turner, "Interpretation of the Decline," pp. 416-417; Newell, *Sources of Mortality Changes*, pp. 106-109; and United Nations, *Foetal, Infant and Early Childhood Mortality*, 1:47-48.

54. M. W. Beaver, "Population, Infant Mortality and Milk," *Population Studies* 27, no. 2 (July 1973):243-254.

55. John E. Gordon, Moises Behar, and Nevin S. Scrimshaw, "Acute Diarrheal Disease in Less Developed Countries," in *Control of Gastrointestinal Diseases* (Washington, D.C.: Pan American Health Organization, 1964), p. 29.

56. During the early decades of the century hardly any dry or canned milk was produced locally. Hence, the figures on imports can reasonably represent the total consumption of these goods. For later decades this was not the case, since many dairy-related industries experienced substantial growth. The figures on per capita consumption of milk substitutes from 1902 to 1927 are taken from República de Cuba, *Comercio Exterior* (Havana, 1902-1958).

Year	Per Capita Consumption (Kilograms)	Year	Per Capita Consumption (Kilograms)
1902	1.97	1915	6.12
1903	1.84	1916	5.99
1904	2.32	1917	6.02
1905	3.18	1918	6.33
1906	3.87	1919	6.31
1907	4.65	1920	7.74
1908	3.89	1921	6.20
1909	4.08	1922	5.81
1910	5.68	1923	6.43
1911	6.06	1924	6.40
1912	5.66	1925	6.24
1913	6.14	1926	6.26
1914	5.97	1927	6.36

During the depression, the imports of canned and dry milk were greatly reduced, in some years by almost 100 percent. The figures, however, are difficult to interpret, since national production of foodstuffs was by then beginning to be emphasized for reasons noted earlier. By the late 1940s and early 1950s, when economic conditions had improved, the figures on national consumption of canned and dry milk on a per capita basis (estimated from data on imports and national production) attained levels similar to those observed during the early 1920s.

57. O. Andrew Collver, *Birth Rates in Latin America: New Estimates of Historical Trends and Fluctuations* (Berkeley: Institute of International Studies, University of California, 1965). The estimated values of the birth rates for Cuba are as follows:

Period	Birth Rate	Age-Standardized Birth Rate
1900-04	44.6	43.6
1905-09	47.4	46.3
1910-14	44.7	47.1
1915-19	40.7	46.0
1920-24	36.7	41.6
1925-29	32.9	35.7
1930-34	31.3	32.5
1935-39	30.9	30.7
1940-44	31.9	30.3
1945-49	30.0	28.9

58. Preston, Keyfitz, and Schoen, *Causes of Death*, p. 7.

59. Ibid., p. 7.

60. Sam Shapiro, Edward R. Schlesinger, and Robert E. L. Nesbitt, Jr., have indicated that during the influenza pandemic of 1918, and during the next two years, when influenza remained epidemic, the maternal mortality rate in the United States skyrocketed (*Infant, Perinatal, Maternal, and Childhood Mortality in the United States*, Vital and Health Statistics Monograph, American Public Health Association [Cambridge, Mass.: Harvard University Press, 1968], p. 144). A similar circumstance may help to explain, at least partially, the significant increase in the age-sex-standardized rate of maternal mortality in Havana in 1919.

61. A large maternity hospital sponsored by the municipality was built between 1910 and 1920. Many private clinics and mutualist associations also began offering services to pregnant women. In addition, many of the public hospitals had maternity wards. In the period after 1931, not only did the sulfonamides and antibiotics become available, but improvements were also made in surgical techniques and anesthesia.

62. See Shapiro, Schlesinger, and Nesbitt, *Infant, Perinatal, Maternal, and Childhood Mortality*, pp. 25-30, and 41-46, for a discussion of these problems.

63. Jorge I. Domínguez, *Cuba: Order and Revolution* (Cambridge, Mass.: Harvard University Press, Belknap Press, 1978), p. 52.

64. Ibid., pp. 72-76.

65. Foreign Policy Association, *Problems of the New Cuba* (New York: J. J. Little & Co., 1935); Lowry Nelson, *Rural Cuba* (1950; reprint ed., New York: Octagon Books, 1970); and Agrupación Católica Universitaria, "Encuesta de trabajadores rurales, 1956-57," *Economía y Desarrollo*, no. 12 (July-August 1972), pp. 188-213.

Chapter 7. The Mortality Decline in Cuba after 1953

1. Wyatt MacGaffey and Clifford R. Barnett, *Cuba, Its People, Its Society, Its Culture* (1962; reprint ed., Westport, Conn.: Greenwood Press, 1974), pp. 73-84.

2. Cuban Economic Research Project, *A Study on Cuba* (Coral Gables, Fla.: University of Miami, 1965), p. 621.

3. Ross Danielson, *Cuban Medicine* (New Brunswick, N. J.: Transaction Books, 1979), pp. 119-121.

4. Some questions could be raised about the dependability of this estimate, however, since it was derived by an interpolation procedure using data from around 1953 to 1970. This period is too long, so it is possible that interpolating may conceal significant changes in the secular trend (Alfonso Farnos Morejón, *Cuba: Tablas de mortalidad estimadas por sexo. Período 1955-70,* Estudios Demográficos, series 1, no. 8 (Universidad de la Habana, December 1976).

5. For a discussion of this perspective, see Barent F. Landstreet, *Cuban Population Issues in Historical and Comparative Perspective*, Latin American Studies Program, Dissertation series, no. 75 (Ithaca, N.Y.: Cornell University, 1976), pp. 121-129. Landstreet is cautious in his interpretation and recognizes that biases in the data may be responsible for the observed trend. Jorge Domínguez seems oblivious to potential problems of demographic data (*Cuba: Order and Revolution* [Cambridge, Mass.: Harvard University Press, Belknap Press, 1978], p. 139).

6. Gerardo González and associates agree with my conclusion that no valid interpretation of the secular trend of mortality changes during most of the sixties can be made on the basis of these series (Gerardo González, Germán Correa, Margarita M. Errazuriz, and Raúl Tapia, "Estrategia de desarrollo y transición demográfica: El caso de Cuba," unpublished [Santiago, Chile: Centro Latinoamericano de Demografía, 1978], p. 3:23). It appears that only by 1968 was death registration complete (Ministerio de Salud Pública, *Cuba: Organización de los servicios y nivel de salud* [Havana, 1974], p. 69).

7. It has been claimed that the deterioration of the economy resulted from the exodus of skilled technical and managerial personnel, the American economic blockade of Cuba, serious productivity losses, economic planning mistakes, and disruptions caused by the transformation of the capitalist economy into a socialist one.

8. Carmelo Mesa-Lago, "Economic Policies and Growth," in *Revolutionary Change in Cuba*, ed. Carmelo Mesa-Lago (Pittsburgh, Pa.: University of Pittsburgh Press, 1971), p. 331.

9. An evaluation of Cuba's educational reform is found in Martin Carnoy and Jorge Wertheim, *Cuba: Economic Change and Education Reform, 1955-1974,* World Bank Staff Working Paper, no. 317 (January 1979).

10. It was estimated that in 1970 Cuba's adequate-housing deficit was 1,044,621 units, about 600,000 in urban areas, with the balance in rural areas (Junta Central de Planificación, *La situación de la vivienda en Cuba en 1970 y su evolución perspectiva* [Havana: Editorial ORBE, 1976], p. 56). This deficit, because of population growth, deterioration of the housing stock, and a low rate of housing construction since 1959, was greater than the one estimated for 1959, 655,000 units

(Maruja Acosta and Jorge E. Hardoy, *Urban Reform in Revolutionary Cuba*, Antilles Research Program, Occasional Papers, no. 1 [New Haven, Conn.: 1971], p. 8).

11. Ministerio de Salud Pública, *Cuba*, p. 90.

12. Detailed reviews of how this requirement was met have been provided by Vincente Navarro, "Health, Health Services, and Health Planning in Cuba," *International Journal of Health Services* 2, no. 3 (August 1972):397-432; and by Danielson, *Cuban Medicine*, pp. 127-228. During the early years of the revolution, the number of health personnel (physicians especially) actually declined as many skilled Cubans left the country.

13. Ministerio de Salud Pública, *Cuba*, p. 35.

14. Ibid., p. 49.

15. Ibid., p. 103. These claims made by Cuban authorities are tempered if we note that severe water shortages in Havana, Santiago, and other large Cuban cities are commonplace. To what extent these water shortages have a negative impact on health cannot be determined. There are reports of occasional outbreaks of disease, partly attributed to the deterioration of water-distribution systems in some cities.

16. Junta Central de Planificación, *La situación*, p. 49.

17. Z. Stein and M. Susser, "The Cuban Health System: A Trial of a Comprehensive Service in a Poor Country," *International Journal of Health Services* 2, no. 4 (1972):555.

18. Large outbreaks of dengue fever, a disease transmitted by mosquitoes, in 1977 and 1981 suggest that Cuba is experiencing difficulties similar to those of other countries in controlling the mosquito population. This situation is probably the result of the mosquitoes' resistance to commonly used insecticides. The severity of the 1977 and 1981 dengue outbreaks suggests that the mosquito population in Cuba is very large, and that the Cuban health authorities may have contributed to the development of resistance by overusing insecticides. It is not inconceivable that even malaria may reappear in epidemic proportions, given the high mosquito density (although malaria is not transmitted by the same type of mosquito that transmits dengue fever) and the frequent reports of the appearance of cases of imported malaria in Cuba (see Pan American Health Organization, "Imported Malaria in the Caribbean," *Bulletin of the Pan American Health Organization* 14, no. 4 [1980]:414-415). The mathematics of the epidemiology of malaria is such that a few cases of the disease and a sufficient concentration of mosquitoes can quickly lead to an outbreak (Gordon Harrison, *Mosquitoes, Malaria, and Man: A History of the Hostilities since 1880* [New York: E. P. Dutton, 1978], pp. 205-207).

19. Ministerio de Salud Pública, *Cuba*, p. 90.

20. Rene Dumont believes that both factors were involved (*Cuba: Socialism and Development* [New York: Grove Press, 1970]).

21. Ministerio de Salud Pública, *Cuba*, pp. 113-114. This publication emphasizes that this caloric intake is not an average, but rather the actual personal intake, since each individual receives the same minimum.

22. The use of supplementary dietary allowances to protect the most vulnerable individuals in the face of food shortages may explain why the Cuban government

holds that improvements in average nutritional levels have contributed to better health in the country. Evidence given in Thomas McKeown and C. R. Lowe, *An Introduction to Social Medicine* (Oxford and Edinburgh: Blackwell, 1966), and discussed by William H. McNeill indicates that during the Second World War, when food rationing was used in England and Germany, special food allowances and other measures to improve dietary levels helped maintain (in Germany) or actually improve (in England), health levels (*Plagues and Peoples* [Garden City, N.Y.: Anchor Press, Doubleday, 1976], pp. 286-287).

23. Ministerio de Salud Pública, *Cuba*, pp. 111-112.

24. The use of mass organizations for these purposes has been discussed in various sources. See, for example, Paula E. Hollerbach, "Mortality Related Policies and Trends in Pre- and Post-Revolutionary Cuba," unpublished (New York: Population Council, 1980), pp. 32-35.

25. Dirección de Demografía, Comité Estatal de Estadísticas, *La mortalidad cubana: Sus características, niveles en 1970 y evolución* (Havana, September 1980), p. 85.

26. Dirección de Demografía, Comité Estatal de Estadísticas, and Centro Latinoamericano de Demografía, *Cuba: La mortalidad infantil según variables socioeconómicas y geográficas, 1974* (San José, Costa Rica, 1980), p. 3.

27. Hollerbach, "Mortality Related Policies." During the 1970s, Cuba had one of the world's highest recorded incidences of induced legal abortions (see Paula E. Hollerbach, "Recent Trends in Fertility, Abortion and Contraception in Cuba," *International Family Planning Perspectives* 6, no. 3 [September 1980]:97-106; and Christopher Tietze, *Induced Abortion: 1979* [New York: Population Council, 1979]).

28. Junta Central de Planificación, *Cifras sobre la niñez y la juventud cubanas* (Havana, September 1975).

29. Stein and Susser, "The Cuban Health System," p. 562.

30. These data are in Pan American Health Organization, *Health Conditions in the Americas; 1969-1972* (Washington, D.C., 1974), and *Health Conditions in the Americas; 1973-1976* (Washington, D.C., 1978). I have chosen for comparison the economically more-advanced countries in Latin America, and the United States. The cause-specific rates are given in this source standardized to the age structure of the combined Latin American populations.

31. Puerto Rico probably has rates comparable with, if not lower than those of Cuba.

32. This approach is limited by data inconsistencies from period to period and from country to country. Official government estimates used by the Pan American Health Organization appear to overestimate grossly the life expectancy levels in many Latin American countries. For the earlier dates, whenever possible I have used Eduardo Arriaga's estimates instead of official estimates (*New Life Tables for Latin American Populations in the Nineteenth and Twentieth Centuries*, Population Monograph Series, no. 3 [Berkeley and Los Angeles: University of California Press, 1968]). In general, I believe that for the later date some of the estimates for

Latin American countries are optimistic.

33. This interpretation can only be made very tentatively. In fact, more recent evidence suggests that by 1980 Costa Rica may have attained life expectancy levels comparable to those reached by Cuba for the same date. The implication of the convergence of the estimates for both countries is that, regardless of political or economic system, a heavy emphasis on the provision of health and other services can have a potent impact on health and mortality levels. An important question yet to be answered is how Costa Rica was able to accomplish results similar to Cuba's, although perhaps with a slight lag, without a process as disruptive and costly as the one produced by the Cuban revolution. For recent life expectancy estimates for Costa Rica, see Hugo Villegas and Carlos A. Valverde, "Life Expectancy Trends in Costa Rica," *Bulletin of the Pan American Health Organization* 13, no. 3 (1979):253-256. Uruguay is more of a mystery because, to my knowledge, no dependable recent estimates of life expectancy are available. The severe disruptions experienced by that country during the 1970s probably had an adverse effect on mortality levels.

34. In Argentina a situation contrary to that reported in Cuba exists. It appears that in Argentina the trend of mortality decline has actually been stopped, or perhaps even reversed. Inequalities in regional and social access to health and other services and in income distribution are postulated as causal factors in this instance (see M. Martha Accinelli and Maria S. Muller, "Un hecho inquietante: La evolución reciente de la mortalidad en la Argentina," *Notas de Población* 6, no. 17 [August 1978]:9-18). Similar distributional effects appear to be hindering mortality declines in Brazil (José Alberto M. de Carvalho and Charles H. Wood, "Mortality, Income Distribution, and Rural-Urban Residence in Brazil," *Population and Development Review* 4, no. 3 [September 1978]:405-420).

35. Cole Blasier, "The Soviet Union in the Cuban-American Conflict," in *Cuba in the World*, ed. Cole Blasier and Carmelo Mesa-Lago (Pittsburgh, Pa.: University of Pittsburgh Press, 1979), pp. 37-51. This figure refers exclusively to economic aid; military assistance amounted to at least $2 billion to $3 billion more over the same period. Similar figures for economic assistance (excluding military) to selected countries through bilateral agreements with the United States are presented below. These estimates exclude other assistance received through, for example, multinational lending agencies. The figures are cumulative from 1962 to 1976.

	U.S. Aid (in millions of dollars)
Latin America	
Bolivia	$ 505
Brazil	2,218
Chile	978
Colombia	1,372
Dominican Republic	550
Peru	386
Other Regions	
Israel	1,860
South Korea	2,622
South Vietnam	6,013

By 1979 cumulative Soviet assistance to Cuba had risen to $16.63 billion (National Foreign Assessment Center, *The Cuban Economy: A Statistical Review* [Washington, D.C.: Central Intelligence Agency, 1981], table 35, p. 39).

Chapter 8. Summary and Conclusions
 1. For Jamaica, reservations are in order with regard to the estimates for early years in the series.
 2. John D. Durand, "Comment" (on Samuel H. Preston's "Causes and Consequences of Mortality Declines in Less Developed Countries during the Twentieth Century"), in *Population and Economic Change in Developing Countries*, ed. Richard A. Easterlin (Chicago, Ill.: National Bureau of Economic Research, University of Chicago Press, 1980), pp. 341-347.
 3. Preston suggests that the relative advantage in life expectancy levels observed for Latin American countries in relation to other developing countries may be the result of their special relationships with the United States; he assumes the bilateral health assistance provided by the United States to be responsible. The Cuban findings reported in this study strongly substantiate Preston's hypothesis (Samuel H. Preston, "Causes and Consequences of Mortality Declines in Less Developed Countries during the Twentieth Century," in *Population and Economic Change in Developing Countries*, ed. Richard A. Easterlin [Chicago, Ill.: National Bureau of Economic Research, University of Chicago Press, 1980], pp. 289-341).
 4. The assumed average life expectancy for the beginning of the period is based on the levels estimated by Eduardo Arriaga for other Latin American countries (table 4). It is likely to have been even lower.
 5. Eduardo E. Arriaga and Kingsley Davis, "The Pattern of Mortality Change in Latin America," *Demography* 6, no. 3 (August 1969):223-242.
 6. Samuel H. Preston, "The Changing Relation between Mortality and Level of Economic Development," *Population Studies* 29, no. 2 (July 1975):231-248.
 7. Arriaga and Davis, "The Pattern."
 8. John D. Durand, "Report of Workshop in History of the Mortality Transition," unpublished (Philadelphia: Graduate Group in Demography, University of Pennsylvania, January-May 1975).
 9. Thomas B. Birnberg and Stephen A. Resnick, *Colonial Development: An Econometric Study* (New Haven, Conn.: Yale University Press, 1975).
 10. The countries considered by Birnberg and Resnick in their study were Sri Lanka (1897-1938), Chile (1892-1938), Cuba (1903-1937), Egypt (1891-1937), India (1890-1936), Jamaica (1886-1938), Nigeria (1901-1937), the Philippines (1902-1938), Taiwan (1904-1936), and Thailand (1902-1936). It would be interesting to test whether the countries studied by Birnberg and Resnick but not studied by Durand experienced similar mortality declines at about the same time. The data for Chile in table 25 suggest that the experience of that country was similar. Evidence for British Guiana, another country sharing the characteristics of an export economy, seems to show that that country may have also entered rapid mortality decline at about the same time. See Jay R. Mandle, "The Decline in Mortality in

British Guiana, 1911-1960," *Demography* 7, no. 3 (August 1970):301-315.

11. Birnberg and Resnick, *Colonial Development*, p. 40.

Appendix 1: Evaluation of the Data

1. Vicente de la Guardia, *Estadística demográfica de la Ciudad de la Habana, 1890 and 1891* (Havana, 1891 and 1892); Jorge Le-Roy y Cassá, "Sanitary Improvement in Cuba as Demonstrated by Statistical Data," *Sanidad y Beneficencia* 8, nos. 4-5 (October-November 1912):507-512, and idem, "Sanitation in Cuba: Its Progress," *Sanidad y Beneficencia*, 10, nos. 1-2 (July-August 1913):240-261.

2. Francisco Llaca y Argudín, *Legislación sobre el registro del estado civil en Cuba* (Havana: Rambla, Bouza y Cía., 1930), pp. 321-324.

3. Fernando González Q. y Jorge Debasa, *Cuba: Evaluación y ajuste del censo de 1953 y las estadísticas de nacimientos y defunciones entre 1943 y 1958. Tabla de mortalidad por sexo, 1952-54*, series C, no. 124 (Santiago, Chile: Centro Latinoamericano de Demografía, 1970), p. 5. It may be presumed that these difficulties had to do with the location of the registration offices, costs involved, etc.

4. O. Andrew Collver, *Birth Rates in Latin America: New Estimates of Historical Trends and Fluctuations*, (Berkeley: Institute of International Studies, University of California, 1965).

5. González Q. and Debasa, *Cuba: Evaluación y ajuste del censo.*

6. From 1902 to 1931, 1,259,864 aliens entered the country. One source has estimated that the net contribution amounted to 700,000 individuals (see Cuban Economic Research Project, *A Study on Cuba* [Coral Gables, Fla.: University of Miami, 1965], p. 199). Collver assumes the net contribution to be close to 623,000 between 1900 and 1930. Although the difference between the two estimates is not unduly large, it is sufficient to cast some suspicion.

7. During most of the period (1900 to about 1930), legal migrants were required to enter the country exclusively through the ports of Havana and Santiago (barring occasional relaxation of the rules), partly due to sanitary considerations (the location of the immigrant-admitting stations). However, it was noted at the time that substantial numbers of illegal migrants were entering the country through other ports generally situated closer to the sugar mills where the migrants went to work. Most of these migrants originated from Puerto Rico, Haiti, the Dominican Republic, and Jamaica (see "El problema de la inmigración clandestina," *Sanidad y Beneficencia* 27, no. 2 [February 1917]:140-141).

8. Collver, *Birth Rate*, pp. 31-32, n. 5.

9. Up to the time of the 1940 constitution, the native-born children of parents having foreign citizenship were automatically considered to have the nationality of their parents. On reaching the age of twenty-one, the native-born children of foreign parents were allowed, if they chose, to become Cuban citizens. The 1940 constitution changed the jus sanguinis determination of citizenship to one of jus soli. The effect on the size of the population with foreign citizenship was enormous. In 1931, 443,197 foreign citizens of Cuban birth were enumerated in the census; in

1943, only 2,488 (República de Cuba, *1943 Census* [Havana, n.d.], p. 747). We can surmise the effect on the estimates of confusing citizenship with place of birth. It remains to be established whether or not, in fact, Collver did so.

10. Two different aspects of the quality of registration of births and deaths in Cuba may be considered as possible sources of bias in registration. The most obvious is simple underregistration. The other, although resulting from the same cause, may multiply the deficiencies: since births in Cuba could legally be registered within the first year after birth, and since infant mortality rates were probably high, many infant deaths (in addition to stillbirths) were neither reported as births nor as deaths. The circularity in Collver's reasoning can best be conveyed by quoting his remarks:

Death registration has been considerably better [than birth registration], running about ninety percent complete and showing a reasonable pattern of variation. In view of this it appears that the age distribution of registered deaths can be accepted as representative of the age distribution of all deaths in Cuba. One shortcoming of the registered deaths is that, in accordance with the Napoleonic Code, infants dying before registration of birth were not recorded. Some correction is needed for this omission, but it is difficult to say how much. Since it is well established that there are widely different patterns of infant and child mortality, we have no basis for estimating infant deaths from deaths of older children . . . . For the present estimates, the age distribution of deaths is accepted as given [p. 111].

11. The quality of six censuses over half a century should vary more than that of two censuses taken ten years apart, and the impact of international migration was much reduced during the later part of the period. Also, the ten-year census interval of 1943-53 facilitated the application of diverse estimating techniques that require the grouping of data in five-year age classes without having to rely on cumbersome and often questionable adjustment procedures for intercensal periods shorter or longer than ten years (or, at least, not in five-year multiples). This is especially so in populations experiencing large flows and ebbs of migration.

12. The comparison countries were selected by looking at geographical proximity, similar levels in certain economic and demographic indicators, and the existence of dependable statistics.

13. The proximity of Jamaica and Cuba, their similar climates, and their basically identical economies suggest that their mortality experiences at the beginning of the century were not very different.

14. República de Cuba, *Censo 1953* (Havana, n.d.), p. xxxiii.

15. The data for 1953 were published in 1958 and 1959.

16. Dirección de Demografía, Comité Estatal de Estadísticas, *La mortalidad cubana: sus características, niveles en 1970 y evolución* (Havana, September 1980).

17. Vincente Navarro, "Health, Health Services, and Health Planning in Cuba," *International Journal of Health Services* 2, no. 3 (November 1972):403.

18. A brief review of the studies that have evaluated the quality of these censuses may be found in Centro Latinoamericano de Demografía (San José), Dirección de Demografía, Comité Estatal de Estadísticas (Cuba), "Proyección de la población

cubana 1950-2000, nivel nacional: Metodología y resultados" (Havana, August 1978), pp. 3-13.

19. Junta Central de Planificación, *Censo de población y viviendas 1970* (Havana: Editorial ORBE, 1975), pp. vii-xv.

Appendix 3: The Life Tables for Havana and Cuba

1. I estimated them with the life-table program found in Nathan Keyfitz and Wilhelm Flieger, *Population: Facts and Methods of Demography* (San Francisco, Cal.: W. H. Freeman & Co., 1971), pp. 127-157.

2. Rodolfo Mezquita, *Cuba: Estimación de la mortalidad por sexo. Tabla de vida para los períodos 1919-31 y 1931-43*, series C, no. 121 (Santiago, Chile: Centro Latinoamericano de Demografía, March 1970); and Fernando González Q. and Jorge Debasa, *Cuba: Evaluación y ajuste del censo de 1953 y las estadísticas de nacimientos y defunciones entre 1943 y 1958. Tabla de mortalidad por sexo, 1952-54*, series C, no. 124 (Santiago, Chile: Centro Latinoamericano de Demografía, June 1970).

3. Junta Central de Planificación, *La esperanza o expectativa de vida* (Havana, 1974), pp. 35-36.

4. The technique used is described in United Nations, *Methods of Estimating Basic Demographic Measures from Incomplete Data*, ST/SOA/series A/42 (New York, 1967).

5. Ansley J. Coale and Paul Demeny, *Regional Model Life Tables and Stable Populations* (Princeton, N. J.: Princeton University Press, 1966).

6. Jeremiah M. Sullivan, "The Influence of Cause-Specific Mortality Conditions on the Age Pattern of Mortality with Special Reference to Taiwan," *Population Studies* 27, no. 1 (March 1973):135-158.

7. Mezquita, the CELADE investigator who derived the life tables, does not note that the age distribution of the foreign-born whites is given in all three censuses. It would seem safer to assume that the total foreign-born population had approximately these same age distributions, since the foreign-born whites acounted for a very large share of all the migrants.

8. United Nations, *Methods for Population Projections by Sex and Age*, Manual 3, ST/SOA/series A, Population Studies, no. 25 (New York, 1956). The age schedule given in table 47, p. 64, was used in the case of immigration, and that in table 48, p. 65, in the case of emigration.

9. See, for example, *Population Bulletin* of the United Nations, no. 6 (1963), p. 60; and Samuel H. Preston, *Mortality Patterns in National Populations with Special Reference to Recorded Causes of Death* (New York: Academic Press, 1976), pp. 120-159.

10. See Appendix 1 for O. Andrew Collver, *Birth Rates in Latin America: New Estimates of Historical Trends and Fluctuations*, (Berkeley: Institute of International Studies, University of California, 1965).

11. Elio Velázquez and Lázaro Toirao, *Cuba: Tablas de mortalidad estimadas por sexo, para los años calendarios terminados en cero y cinco durante el período*

1900-1950, Estudios Demográficos, series 1, no. 3 (Havana: Universidad de la Habana, July 1975). It should be noted that the life tables estimated in this study are partly based on the biased life tables for 1925 and 1937, evaluated in this Appendix; therefore, they present corresponding errors.

Appendix 4: Classification of Causes of Death
  1. Samuel H. Preston, Nathan Keyfitz, and Robert Schoen, *Causes of Death* (New York: Seminar Press, 1972), pp. 4-8.

Bibliography of Sources
Not Cited in Text

Bonachea, Rolando E., and Nelson P. Valdés, eds. *Cuba in Revolution*. New York: Doubleday & Co., 1972.

de Castro y Bachiller, Raimundo. *Centenario del nacimiento del Dr. Jorge Le-Roy y Cassá*. Cuaderno de Historia de la Salud Pública. Havana, 1968.

Centro de Estudios Demográficos. *La población de Cuba*. Committee for International Coordination of National Research in Demography series. Havana: Instituto Cubano del Libro, 1976.

Dirección Central de Estadística, Junta Central de Planificación. *Análisis de las características demográficas de la población cubana. Censo de población y viviendas de 1970: Anticipo de datos por muestreo*. Havana, 1973.

Durand, John D. "Demographic Transition." *International Population Conference Proceedings*, Sidney, 1967, pp. 32-45.

Dyer, Donald R. "Urbanism in Cuba." *Geographical Review* 47, no. 2 (April 1957):224-233.

Hernández, Roberto E. "La atención médica en Cuba hasta 1958." *Journal of Inter-American Studies* 11, no. 4 (October 1969):533-557.

Jenks, Leland Hamilton. *Our Cuban Colony: A Study in Sugar*. St. Clair Shores, Mich.: Scholarly Press, 1972.

Junta Nacional de Sanidad y Beneficencia. *Escarlatina, instrucciones populares para evitar su contagio y propagación*. Havana, 1905.

Junta Superior de Sanidad. *Informe anual sanitario y demográfico de la República de Cuba*. 7 vols. Havana, 1902-1908.

_____. *Informe anual sanitario y demográfico del término municipal de la Habana*. 7 vols. Havana, 1902-1908.

Lebowitz, Michael D. "Influence of Urbanization and Industrialization on Birth and Death Rates." *Social Biology* 20, no. 1 (March 1973):89-102.

Le Riverend Brusone, Julio. "Historia económica." In *Historia de la nación cubana*, ed. Ramiro Guerra y Sánchez et al.,pp. 7:151-244; 9:287-396. Havana:

Editorial Historia de la Nación Cubana, 1952.

McKeown, Thomas. "Medicine and World Population." In *Public Health and Population Change*, ed. Mindell C. Sheps and Jeanne Clare Ridley, pp. 25-40. Pittsburgh, Pa.: University of Pittsburgh Press, 1965.

_____, and R. G. Brown. "Medical Evidence Related to English Population Changes in the Eighteenth Century." *Population Studies* 9, no. 2 (November 1955):119-141.

Martínez Fortún, Ortelio, and Mariano Martín Díaz. "Las estadísticas sanitarias en Cuba." In *Proceedings of the Eighth American Scientific Congress*, Washington, D.C., 1943, vol. 3.

Mesa-Lago, Carmelo. "Availability and Reliability of Statistics in Socialist Cuba." *Latin American Research Review* 4, no. 1 (Spring 1969):53-91; and 4, no. 2 (Summer 1969):47-81.

_____. *Cuba in the 1970s: Pragmatism and Institutionalization*. Albuquerque: University of New Mexico Press, 1974.

Oficina de Estudios del Plan de Seguridad Social. *Condiciones económicas y sociales de la República de Cuba: Informe preparado por la Oficina de Estudios del Plan de Seguridad Social*. Havana: Editorial Lex, 1944.

Oshima, H. T. "A New Estimate of the National Income and Product of Cuba in 1953." *Food Research Institute Studies* 2, no. 3 (November 1961):213-227.

Pérez de la Riva, Juan. "La population de Cuba y ses problèmes." *Population* 22, no. 1 (January-February 1967):99-110.

Preston, Samuel H. "Influence of Cause of Death Structure on Age-Patterns of Mortality." In *Population Dynamics*, ed. T. N. E. Greville, pp. 201-250. New York: Academic Press, 1972.

Shryock, Henry S., and Jacob S. Siegel. *The Methods and Materials of Demography*. Washington, D.C.: U.S. Government Printing Office, 1975.

Stolnitz, George J. "A Century of International Mortality Trends. *Population Studies* 9, no. 1 (July 1955):24-55; and 10, no. 1 (July 1956):17-42.

_____. "International Mortality Trends: Some Main Facts and Implications. In *The Population Debate*, pp. 1:220-236. New York: United Nations, 1975.

Thorning, Joseph F. "Social Medicine in Cuba. *The Americas* 1, no. 4 (April 1945): 440-455.

Vallin, Jacques. "La mortalité dans les pays du tiers monde: Evolution et perspectives." *Population* 23, no. 5 (September-October 1968):845-868.

Index

Abortion, 110
Age structure, 11, 66
Agricultural revolution, 5
Aid, foreign, 117-118
American Public Health Association, 81
Antibiotics, 51, 81, 86, 88, 124, 129
Antiseptic packages, for care of umbilicus of newborn, 82, 124
Aqueducts, 41, 44-45, 83, 108
Argentina, 20-21, 112-113, 119, 156, 158
Arriaga, Eduardo E., 8, 20, 22, 116, 130-131

BCG vaccine, 68-69
Beaver, M. W., 90
Behm, Hugo, 66
Benenson, Abram S., 77
Biases, estimation, 18
Birth rate, 5-6, 13, 91, 104
Bourdé, Guy, 13
Brazil, 20
Breast feeding, 88
Buenos Aires, 20
Burial regulations, 32

Camagüey (city), 44
Canada, 113

Causes of death: accidents and violence, 57, 62, 98; cardiovascular disease, 9, 57, 63, 66, 101, 124-125; cholera, 12, 25-27, 132; cirrhosis of the liver, 91; degenerative diseases, 9, 57, 63, 112, 125; diabetes, 91; diarrheal diseases, 9, 45, 57, 62, 66, 101, 111-112, 123, 125; diphtheria, 27, 30, 62, 82, 123; dysentery, 25, 80; endocarditis, acute, 84; enteric fevers, 25, 27, 30, 62-63, 80-81, 123; infancy, diseases of, 57; infectious and parasitic diseases, 7, 9, 25, 27, 56-57, 62-63, 66, 73-84, 112, 123, 125; influenza, bronchitis, pneumonia, 5, 9, 15, 57, 62-63, 86, 119, 125; intestinal parasites, 83-84; malaria, 5, 7, 27, 30, 33, 51, 57, 74-77, 101-102, 109, 119, 123, 125, 131; malnutrition, 7, 28, 47, 80 (*see also* Nutrition); measles, 57, 62, 72, 76, 80, 113; meningitis, 57, 62, 81; nephritis, 91; poliomyelitis, 113; rheumatic fever, 84; scarlet fever, 82; smallpox, 7, 12, 27, 30, 32, 76-77, 119, 123, 129; stillbirth, 96; suicide, 96; syphilis, 82; tetanus, 27, 30, 57, 62, 81-82, 123; tuberculosis, 9, 27-28,

Causes of death (*continued*) 30, 33, 56, 57, 63, 66-73, 101, 123-124; tumors, malignant and benign, 56, 63, 124-125; whooping cough, 77; yellow fever, 12, 25-27, 30, 32-33, 81, 123, 131
Censuses, 11; data, 144; quality of, 12
Centro Latinoamericano de Demografía (CELADE), 16, 19-20, 104, 144, 154, 156, 158
Chemotherapy, 8, 68, 69, 83
Chile, 66, 119, 122-123, 131, 139-141
China, 25
Civil unrest, effects on mortality of, 98
Coale, Ansley J., 154, 156
Collver, O. Andrew, 91, 135-151, 144, 163
Comisión Económica para América Latina (CEPAL, ECLA), 38
Conditions: economic, 3-4, 8, 25, 33, 35, 37-38, 83, 91, 96, 98, 100-101, 103-104, 117, 123, 125-130; political, 35, 37-38, 48, 101, 117, 126-129; sanitary, 13, 25-26, 28, 36, 80, 105, 108-109 (*see also* Public health); social, 3-4, 35, 98, 100-101; socioeconomic, 6; working, 67
Contagion, 67
Contraception, 110
Costa Rica, 20-21, 113, 119, 122, 140-141
Cuba, national agencies of: Comité Estatal de Estadísticas, 144; Dirección de Demografía, 19; Junta Central de Planificación (JUCE-PLAN), 19, 116; Junta Nacional del Censo, 12; National Bank of, 38; National Bureau of Statistics and Information, 68; National Council of Tuberculosis, 68

Data adjustments, 13

Death rate, 5, 6, 11-13, 15, 27-28, 32; age-sex-specific, 53-54; age-sex-standardized, cause-specific, 55-56, 58; cause-specific, 27, 30; provincial, 15; standardized, 11, 16
Death registration, 11-12, 16, 104, 112; completeness of, 134-144; legal and classificatory aspects of, 133-134. *See also* Underregistration, of deaths
Death statistics, adjustments to: City of Havana, 142-143, 149; revolutionary Cuba, 143-144
Debasa, Jorge, 19, 116, 136-141
Demeny, Paul, 154, 156
Denmark, 121
Development, socioeconomic, 9
Disease control: international efforts at, 131; technology of, 33
Diseases. *See* Causes of death
Disease vectors, control of, 33
Dominican Republic, 20
Durand, John D., 5, 122, 131

Economic growth, 8, 25, 35-36, 38, 124, 131
Education, 73, 80, 117, 124, 129-130. *See also* Literacy
Employment, policies, 105
England and Wales, 8, 73, 77, 82, 88
Epidemics, 7, 12-13, 25-26, 28
Europe, 26
Expeditionary force, Spanish, 13

Facilities, medical, 48, 50-51, 68-69, 73, 83, 93, 96, 103, 105-108, 110, 112-113, 124-125, 129
Famine, 7, 13
Fertility, 27, 84, 93, 96, 132
First World War, 131
Foreign Policy Association, 50

Germ theory of disease, 8

González Q., Fernando, 19, 116, 136-141
Great Depression, 18, 38, 73, 101, 123-124
Guatemala, 119
Guyana (British Guiana), 7, 51, 139-141

Haiti, 76
Homicides, 96
Housing conditions, 41, 44, 67, 73, 83, 90, 105
Hygiene, personal, 90

Immigration, 15, 25-26, 48, 50, 76-77, 98, 137, 156-158
Immunization, 7-8
Income: distribution of, 8, 38, 128-129, 131; level, 8; national, 40; per capita, 38-39, 48, 103, 131; redistribution of, 105, 125
Industrial Revolution, 7
Infant mortality, 104, 110, 117; endogenous causes of, 96
Inoculation, 7. See also Diseases: smallpox
Insecticides, 8, 33, 51, 76-77, 102, 125
International Bank for Reconstruction and Development (World Bank), 37
International List of Causes of Death, 56, 134-135, 167-171
Interrelationship, socioeconomic and demographic, 4
Investment, foreign, 36-37, 123

Jamaica, 76, 113, 119, 122, 131, 139-141
Japan, 7, 122, 131

Keyfitz, Nathan, 84, 167-168
Knight, Franklin W., 27

Labor, indentured, 25

Latin America, 8, 20, 33, 131
Life expectancy, 4, 18-20, 22, 112
Life tables, 11, 16, 18, 55; model, 154, 156
Literacy, 45-46, 90, 105. See also Education
Living conditions, 38, 86, 98, 100-101; rural-urban differentials in, 4, 102, 105

McKeown, Thomas, 7-8, 54, 73, 77, 82, 88
Matanzas clay, effect on malaria prevalence of, 76
Medical and public health developments, 5-9, 35, 37, 51, 68, 82-83, 96, 102-103, 113, 123-125, 130-131
Medicine, preventive, 105-107
Mexico, 119, 122
Military occupation of Cuba, U.S., 13, 15
Milk, canned and dry, 90, 124; pasteurization of, 67-68, 90
Mortality: by age, 9, 53-55; colonial, 26; maternal (complications of pregnancy), 57, 110, 125; old age, 63; perinatal, 110; premodern, 12; rural, 26, 46-47; slave, 27; transition, 6, 9, 127-128; urban, 46-47
Mortality decline: contribution of different causes to, 60; direct mechanisms of, 126-131; economic costs of, 117-118; mediating mechanisms of, 126-129; models of, 6-7, 21, 122-123; relative impact of determinants of, 126-131
Mosquitoes, 7, 32, 74, 76-77
Mutualist health associations, 50, 83, 103, 124

Nicaragua, 20
Norway, 122
Nutrition, 8, 33, 47-48, 67, 73, 77,

Nutrition (*continued*) 80, 86, 88, 90-91, 101, 109, 112-113, 124-125, 129-130. *See also* Diseases: malnutrition

Omran, Abdel, 6, 21

Panama, 20
Pan American Health Organization (PAHO), 115-116
Pandemic, influenza (1918), 88
Paraguay, 20
Pestilence, 13
Physician, availability of, 48, 50; population per, 48, 106-107
Platt Amendment, 35-37, 123
Population: age composition of, 16; estimates of, 145-149; growth of, 5-6; sex composition of, 16; size of, 13
Prebisch, Raúl, 38
Preston, Samuel H., 8-9, 57, 66, 84, 91, 131, 167-168
Public health: efforts at, 36, 45, 109, 117; and sanitary reforms, 4, 8, 32-33, 90, 101, 119, 126-130; policies, in revolutionary Cuba, 105-106
Puerto Rico, 113

Quarantine, regulations, 32, 76-77
Quinine, 76-77

Record, R. G., 77, 88
Records, ecclesiastical, 13
Reforms, revolutionary Cuba: economic and social, in, 112; institutional, 113
Rice, consumption per capita of, 47-48. *See also* Nutrition
Rockefeller Foundation, 74

Sanitary reform movement, 32
Sanitation, environmental, 33, 88, 124, 129

Santa Maria del Rosario (city), 13
Santiago de Cuba (city), 44-45
Schoen, Robert, 84, 167-168
Second World War, 7, 20-21, 38, 46, 51, 66, 73, 76, 101-102, 123, 125, 130
Sewage, 41-42, 44-45
Slaves, 25-26
Social class, 4
Socialist revolution, 4, 10, 104-118, 125, 128
Soviet Union, 117
Spain, 28
Spanish-American War, 4, 13, 21, 119. *See also* War of Independence
Sri Lanka (Ceylon), 7, 51, 119, 122, 131
Statistics, health, 32
Stein, Z., 111-112
Sugar, 25, 28, 37-38, 41, 47, 123-125
Sulfonamides, 51, 86, 88, 125, 130
Susser, M., 111-112
Sweden, 122

Taiwan, 119, 122, 131
Thomas, Hugh, 12-13, 26
Trade, international, 25-26, 37-38, 40, 48, 91, 102, 126, 131
Transition, demographic, 6
Trinidad and Tobago, 113
Turner, R. D., 77, 88

Ulcers, of stomach and duodenum, 91
Underregistration, of deaths, 12-13, 16, 69
United Nations, 116, 158
United States, 4, 26, 28, 33, 35-37, 47, 68, 80-81, 83, 101, 112, 119, 123, 125, 126; Bureau of the Census, 22; War Department, 15
Urbanization, 44-46, 132
Uruguay, 112-113

Venezuela, 20
Virulence, 7

War of Independence, 12-13, 28. *See
  also* Spanish-American War
Water supplies, 41, 43-45, 90, 108,
  129

Welfare, 3, 101, 117-118
World Bank (International Bank for
  Reconstruction and Development),
  37

Yellow Fever Commission, 32